Foundations of Healthcare Ethics

Theory to practice

In order to provide the highest level of care to their patients and clients, health professionals need a sound knowledge and understanding of healthcare ethics. *Foundations of Healthcare Ethics: Theory to practice* focuses on the philosophical concepts that underpin contemporary ethical discourse for health professionals, and arms both students and professionals with the knowledge to tackle situations of moral uncertainty in clinical practice.

The text has been specially written to provide an in-depth study of the theoretical foundations of healthcare ethics. It covers a range of normative ethical theories, from virtue ethics to utilitarianism, while also investigating their application to contemporary issues in healthcare and society. The book provides opportunities for self-directed learning, and also presents questions and case studies to facilitate engagement and discussion.

Foundations of Healthcare Ethics: Theory to practice provides both students and professionals with an understanding of the philosophy governing healthcare ethics in order to help them provide a better level of care to all patients and clients.

Jānis (John) T. Ozoliņš is Professor of Philosophy at the Australian Catholic University and permanent Honorary Fellow, University of Latvia.

Joanne Grainger is a lecturer and healthcare ethicist in the School of Nursing, Midwifery and Paramedicine at the Australian Catholic University.

Foundations of Healthcare Ethics

Theory to practice

Edited by

Jānis T. Ozoliņš & Joanne Grainger

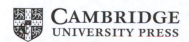

CAMBRIDGE
UNIVERSITY PRESS

477 Williamstown Road, Port Melbourne, VIC 3207, Australia

Cambridge University Press is part of the University of Cambridge.

It furthers the University's mission by disseminating knowledge in the pursuit of education, learning and research at the highest international levels of excellence.

www.cambridge.org
Information on this title: www.cambridge.org/9781107639645

First published 2015

Cover designed by Sardine Design
Typeset by Integra Software Services Pvt. Ltd
Printed in Singapore by C.O.S. Printers Pte Ltd

A catalogue record for this publication is available from the British Library

A Cataloguing-in-Publication entry is available from the catalogue of the National Library of Australia at www.nla.gov.au

ISBN 978-1-107-63964-5 Paperback

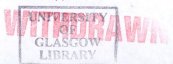

In memory of Jacob Jānis Ozoliņš (1981–2013) and for my family.

Jānis (John) Ozoliņš

For my parents Jill and Len Grainger, whose love and extraordinary work ethic have both inspired and enabled me to choose the career path of fostering a culture of life in healthcare.

Joanne Grainger

Foreword

'My Hippocratic oath tells me to cut a gangrenous appendix out of the human body. The Jews are the gangrenous appendix of mankind. That's why I cut them out.' So explained one of the doctors working in a Nazi death camp during World War II. He thought the procedures he carried out at Auschwitz were justifiable on *medical* grounds. Killing Jews, Gypsies, Catholics, the mentally and physically disabled, homosexuals and other vulnerable people by various methods – including starvation, lethal injection or poisoning with carbon monoxide – furthered Hitler's aim of cleansing the gene pool and ensuring the Aryan race's dominion over all other races (Cook, 2014, citing Lifton, 2000: 232).

Unfortunately, the Allied Powers do not escape culpability for the misuse of science and medicine. In recent years, reports have emerged of unethical medical experiments conducted by the Americans in Guatemala after World War II. Dr John Cutler, who eventually rose to be US Assistant Surgeon-General, led this project and was associated with a parallel one in Tuskegee, Alabama. To study the course of sexually transmitted diseases and the effect of penicillin, the US Public Health Service deliberately infected soldiers, prostitutes, prisoners and mental patients with syphilis without their knowledge or consent. The 1997 film *Miss Evers' Boys* brought the Alabama part of that story to public attention, and led to an apology by President Bill Clinton. But it was not until 2011 that a Commission of Inquiry reported the full horror of the Guatemalan phase of the study: instead of the few dozen victims previously acknowledged, there were in fact at least two thousand healthy men deliberately infected, many of whom in turn infected their wives and children. Instead of being treated with penicillin, they were all given placebos so the researchers could observe the course of the disease as it took its terrible toll on their bodies and minds, and eventually killed them (Presidential Commission for the Study of Bioethical Issues, 2011).

Such research is obviously monstrous. But what shocked many people was that it was still going on in 1970s America. The international legal instruments to guarantee human rights and the World Medical Association's declarations to ensure a high standard of medical ethics that came after the terrible Nazi experiments of the 1930s and 1940s were supposed to prevent such things from ever occurring again. No doctor would ever again intentionally torture or kill, and no government or profession would ever again sponsor such practices. For sensitive students, health professionals, lawyers and ethicists – such as those who may read this textbook – this must raise deep questions. Why would some people fail to abide by the most basic principles of morality, known not only to the world's great religions, but also to sound medicine and nursing, the common law and good secular philosophy?

Unfortunately, atrocities in the name of medicine or research cannot be confined to the garbage bin of history. Richard Dawkins, prominent scientist and evangelist for atheism, claimed recently that not only are parents free to abort children with Down syndrome: they actually have a moral obligation to do so. This comment followed in the wake of revelations that some surrogate mothers were refusing to abort children they were carrying on behalf of other couples, who had been found to have Down Syndrome and whose commissioning parents had directed be terminated (Flynn, 2014). Julian Savulescu, an Australian bioethicist at Oxford University, admitted that eugenics is practised all the time in contemporary healthcare, especially through 'search and destroy' pre-natal screening and genetic tests; however, because it is a matter of 'free choice', it is at least rhetorically different from the Nazi eugenics program (cited in Cook, 2014). That said, Dawkins, Savulescu and others believe there is not just a right but a duty to abort the handicapped and a duty to improve the genetic pool where we can. How soon this duty will be sufficiently politically palatable to be made law or medical policy is uncertain, but bioethics will on their view be no barrier to such social trends.

Clearly declarations of moral principle for healthcare practice are important: they offer a basis for professional unity, identity, regulation and education; they allow health professionals to tell themselves and those who entrust themselves to their care that 'this is what we stand for; this is what we will do and not do and why'. They are therefore crucial to the health professional–patient relationship. But such ethics statements are never enough: eternal vigilance is required to ensure they are truly observed, and we need medical practitioners of good character who will actually apply them wisely and consistently. In the struggle for the soul of our culture, the battlegrounds are increasingly hospitals and aged care facilities, parliaments and courts, bureaucracies and academies. If our highest values are to survive and be enacted, healthcare will require students and professionals of intelligence and courage. If healthcare is to be worthy of the reverence and rewards received in our community, if people are to continue to trust health professionals, the practitioners must be principled and virtuous.

We must understand, for instance, what healthcare is for and how its internal goals might reasonably be pursued. The therapeutic and research imperatives to get results 'no matter what'; the technological imperative to pursue the technically possible even if morally troubling; the demands of patients, administrators and financiers; the practitioners' feelings of impotence and fantasies of omnipotence: all can militate against ethics in practice. Doctors and nurses are by no means alone in this. Ethics committees and legal and moral advisers to health institutions can feel pressured to be 'part of the team', getting results no matter what the cost to justice and ethics. Even philosophers and theologians – who should be the experts at raising questions as much as providing answers – can all too easily become window-dressers for the ideologies of the age or the convenience of those they are advising.

Yet ordinary people still look to their professionals to provide not just a high level of technical care but highly ethical care. Here's one reason why. When the best pagan doctors sought to follow Hippocrates or the best Christian doctors the Good Samaritan, when Jews and Muslims brought the wisdom of Maimonides and Avicenna to the West and through the West to the world, when more recent practitioners re-consecrated themselves to the Geneva Declaration, all swore *an oath* – not an employment contract or protocol, but an oath: a prayer and promise to God, or the gods, or whatever people hold most precious. That is a humble act, acknowledging that both goodness and health ultimately come from a source greater than ourselves; that on joining and practising in my profession I am engaging in more than a job, in something more like a God-given 'vocation'. Solemnly to consecrate my life to the service of humanity; to say I will put the life and health of my patients first and always respect their dignity and privacy; to resolve to save and heal and care, never kill or harm or abandon; to promise to honour my teachers and build up my profession: to commit to such things requires all that is best in the human spirit and God's help also.

✳ ✳ ✳

Amy Gutmann, President of the University of Pennsylvania and Chair of the Guatemala Commission, said that the experiments the US government carried out 'should shock the conscience not in spite of their medical context, but precisely because of it'. We rightly expect more of our professionals. We expect our health professionals to be protectors of life and health and dignity.

Although there have been many failures, and although contemporary bio-ethics is in many ways in disarray, all is not lost. In your hands is a textbook that aims to provide our future practitioners with the intellectual resources to be more than mere witchdoctors and hired guns. This work, authored by a number of respected ethicists, theologians and philosophers, provides professionals, students and the general reader with an accessible entrée to the ethics of healthcare, informed by a Catholic intellectual perspective and mostly in accord with that church's bioethical teaching. It is not straitened by a utilitarian ethic that precludes the possibility of absolutes or by deontological ethics that preclude the possibility of questions. It is, rather, open to questions about what healthcare is and what it is for, what a health professional is and what they are for, what a good professional practice is and what sorts of practices might be morally 'shady'. It accepts that central to medical practice are the goals of saving, healing and caring, and principles against killing, harming or abandoning. Though avoiding over-simplifications, it insists that sound practice requires respect for the dignity or inviolability of the human being from conception until natural death.

Rather than diving straight into the ethical conundrums that are the stuff of TV hospital shows or media headlines, this book valuably begins by grounding our reflection in the range of ethical approaches, from 'principlism' to Kantian ethics, empathy and care, virtue ethics and natural law. Exploration of the latter two theories in particular is helpful in providing students with ways of thinking about ethics that build on classical thought and modern declarations, that make sense of what health professionals actually do and aspire to, yet that receive far too little exposure in our culture today. In this regard, Aristotle, Aquinas and the great tradition on the human person, happiness and practical reason get a thorough workout in this volume, and the authors are unafraid to refer appropriately to God and spirituality. This is because healthcare has become not only a battleground for the soul of our culture, as suggested above, but also a place where sensitive and ethical practitioners today must ask for themselves the big questions about what it is to be a good person and live a good life. Put baldly, good nurses and doctors are not merely excellent technicians but also *good*. And so they need the sort of intellectual equipment and moral formation this book proposes.

Building on such philosophical and theological foundations, this book then readies the reader to confront a number of topical ethical issues, such as conceptualising human dignity, conscience and the health professional; the beginning of life; autonomy and consent; the interaction between law and autonomy at the end of life; organ donation and brain death; and issues of justice, health resource-allocation and palliative care for the dying. Thus practitioners and students are provided with a way through the maze of real-life challenges that they are likely to confront.

Foundations of Healthcare Ethics: Theory to practice is an important addition to the library of any student or practitioner who wishes to approach healthcare in ways that are reasonable and compassionate, that accord with the long wisdom of the profession itself and the wider philosophical-theological tradition, and that allow both practitioners and those for whom they care to live 'the good life' to its natural end.

Most Rev. Anthony Fisher OP, Archbishop of Sydney

References

Cook, M. (2014). Lest we forget. *Mercatornet*, 4 September. Retrieved 20 September 2014 from <http://www.mercatornet.com/articles/view/lest_we_forget1>.

Flynn, J. (2014). When babies become commodities: The new eugenics. *Zenit*, 7 September. Retrieved 20 September 2014 from <http://www.zenit.org/en/articles/when-babies-become-commodities>.

Lifton, R. J. (2000). *The Nazi doctors: Medical killing and the psychology of genocide*. New York: Basic Books.

Presidential Commission for the Study of Bioethical Issues (2011). *'Ethically impossible' STD research in Guatemala from 1946 to 1948*. Washington, DC: Presidential Commission.

Contents

List of contributors

Frank Brennan SJ, AO is Professor of Law at the Australian Catholic University and Adjunct Professor at the Australian National University College of Law and National Centre for Indigenous Studies. He was the founding director of Uniya, the Australian Jesuit Social Justice Centre. He is a board member of St Vincent's Health Australia. His book, *Acting on Conscience* (2007), looks at the place of religion in Australian politics and law. The National Trust classified him as a Living National Treasure at the same time as Paul Keating labelled him 'the meddling priest'. In 2009, he chaired the Australian National Human Rights Consultation Committee.

Norman Ford, sdb is a Senior Fellow of Catholic Theological College, and a member of both the Department of Philosophy and the Department of Moral Theology and Canon Law. He lectures in bioethics, and ethical theory and practical issues. He has published extensively in bioethics. Among his recent publications are: *Stem Cells, Science, Medicine, Law and Ethics* (co-authored with Michael Herbert, 2003), *The Prenatal Person: Ethics from Conception to Birth* (2002), *Christian Conscience* (2009) and *Ethical Dilemmas in Assisted Reproductive Technologies* (2011); along with many articles in journals and collections.

Joanne Grainger is a registered nurse, healthcare ethicist and post-graduate course coordinator for the School of Nursing, Midwifery and Paramedicine at the Australian Catholic University (ACU). Currently completing a Doctor of Education at Melbourne University, Joanne also lectures in the area of sports ethics for the Masters of High Performance Sport course at ACU. In 2010, Joanne was awarded the prestigious Edmund Pellegrino Fellowship in Bioethics from Georgetown University in Washington DC, the first registered nurse and Australian to receive this award. Also in 2010, Joanne received the Mary Philippa Brazill Foundation national grant for the development of online healthcare ethics education units specifically for post-graduate nurses and midwives across Australia. In 2012, Joanne was conferred the Australian Catholic University Excellence in Teaching award for her leadership in healthcare ethics education at the university and in the public sphere. She has interests in the scholarship areas of military ethics (in particular the role of nurses in the WWII Nazi euthanasia programs), simulation education pedagogy, and research ethics, and is passionate about the academic work and life of Pope John Paul II.

David G. Kirchhoffer is a Lecturer in Theological Ethics in the School of Theology at the Australian Catholic University's McAuley campus in Banyo, Brisbane. He is a South African who holds degrees in psychology and advanced biology, and theology. He completed his doctorate in theological ethics at the Katholieke Universiteit Leuven, Belgium, and worked as a post-doctoral researcher at the Centre for Biomedical Ethics and Law at the Katholieke Universiteit Leuven. He is the author of *Human Dignity in Contemporary Ethics* (2013) and co-editor of *Being Human: Towards a Theological Anthropology for the 21st Century* (2013).

Patrick McArdle is Associate Professor in Theology and Campus Dean of the Canberra Campus of the Australian Catholic University. He is also Director of the Institute for Catholic Identity and Mission. His primary research is related to Christian anthropology, applying his findings in this field to practical theology and Christian ethics, especially in the field of healthcare. His recent publications, including *Relational Health Care: A Practical Theology of Personhood* (2008), centre on healthcare and Christian anthropology, models of formation for those engaged in ministries and other Church-based activities, and the educational impact of relational personhood.

Brigid McKenna is the Director of the Office of Life, Marriage and Family in the Archdiocese of Hobart, Tasmania. She is a medical practitioner and healthcare ethicist and educator. She has degrees from the University of Tasmania (MBBS) and the John Paul II Institute for Marriage and Family (MBioeth). After several years of medical practice, she became the Director of the Life Office, an agency of the Catholic Archdiocese of Sydney involved in bioethical research, education and public policy. She has also taught at the University of Notre Dame Australia, the Australian Catholic University and the University of Tasmania.

Jānis (John) T. Ozoliņš FHERDSA, FPESA, MACE, Foreign Member of the Latvian Academy of Sciences, is Professor of Philosophy at the Australian Catholic University, permanent Honorary Fellow, Institute of Philosophy and Sociology, University of Latvia, and Inaugural Crawford Miller Visiting Fellow at St. Cross College, Oxford. He is a Fellow of the Higher Education Research and Development Society of Australasia, and a Fellow and former President of the Philosophy of Education Society of Australasia. He is also Reviews Editor of *Educational Philosophy and Theory*, Editor of *Res Disputandae* (formerly *Ethics Education*) and an editorial consultant on a number of international refereed journals. He is Secretary-General of the World Union of Catholic Philosophical Societies, Vice-President of the World Conference of Catholic Institutes of Philosophy (COMIUCAP), Regional Coordinator for Oceania of the Centre for Research in Values and Philosophy and a member of the International Association of Catholic Bioethicists. He has interests in the metaphysics of Aquinas, philosophy of education, social philosophy, research ethics and applied ethics, and has published widely in these areas.

Bernadette Tobin is director of the Plunkett Centre for Ethics, a joint centre of the Australian Catholic University and St Vincent's & Mater Health Sydney. She is Conjoint Associate Professor in the Faculty of Medicine at the University of New South Wales and Conjoint Associate Professor in the Faculty of Health Sciences at the University of Sydney. She is Honorary Ethicist at the Children's Hospital at Westmead, Sydney.

1 Why study healthcare ethics?

Patrick McArdle and Joanne Grainger

Studying any discipline is worthwhile simply for the knowledge it brings and the skills in reasoning that can be learned and honed. For healthcare professionals, study – formal and informal – is part of the vocation: competence and excellence are not benchmarks to be achieved once in a lifetime and then relegated to the shelves, as one might a sporting trophy. Rather, the health professions demand a commitment to lifelong learning. Part of that professional commitment is an awareness of and engagement with the ethics of health and healthcare. The skills of this philosophical discipline are just as vital as clinical skills and the various dimensions of physiological and psychological knowledge that are essential for the work of a healthcare professional.

Why ethics?

Ethics has been an important sub-set of philosophy since the time of the ancient Greeks. For those early philosophers, there were three big questions to be answered by every human being and every society:

- What does it mean to be or to exist?
- How do we know – what is knowledge and how do we go about knowing?
- How should we live – what is a good life?

It is the third of these questions that is the core concern of this book.

Without covering the whole of the history of philosophy or the even history of ethics, it should be noted that across the three millennia since the time of the ancient Greeks, the question of how we should live has been debated and tested in every culture and every age. The debate has covered how societies and cultures should operate and what constitutes the good life at a particular point in time. These questions have been asked by people of all levels of education, responsibility, fields of employment and political persuasions.

In terms of the collection of disciplines that come under the banner of healthcare, there has always been one part of the broad topic of ethics that has been of particular interest – for instance Hippocrates taught his followers that all physicians had to always act to preserve life and alleviate suffering, but also that they must keep confidential anything they heard or saw while with a patient or in their home. In medieval times, the question of the use of bone materials from the dead and from animals to repair skull damage of those injured in war was a significant question. Still later, the use of the early anaesthetic ether to ease birth pains was very controversial in the late nineteenth and early twentieth centuries. It is also fair to note that these discussions established only broad parameters for a separate body of thinking on the ethics of healthcare.

Hippocratic Oath – classical version

I swear by Apollo Physician and Asclepius and Hygieia and Panaceia and all the gods and goddesses, making them my witnesses, that I will fulfil according to my *ability* and *judgment* this oath and *this covenant*:

- To hold him who has taught me this art as equal to my parents and to live my life in partnership with him, and if he is in need of money to give him a share of mine, and to regard his offspring as equal to my brothers in male lineage and to teach them this art – if they desire to learn it – without fee and covenant; to give a share of precepts and oral instruction and all the other learning to my sons and to the sons of him who has instructed me and to pupils who have signed the covenant and have taken an oath according to the medical law, but no one else.
- I will apply *dietetic measures for the benefit of the sick according to my ability and judgment; I will keep them from harm and injustice.*
- I will neither give a deadly drug to anybody who asked for it, nor

will I make a suggestion to this effect. Similarly *I will not give to a woman an abortive remedy.* In purity and holiness I will guard my life and my art.

- *I will not use the knife*, not even on sufferers from stone, but will withdraw in favor of such men as are engaged in this work.
- *Whatever houses I may visit, I will come for the benefit of the sick*, remaining free of all intentional injustice, of all mischief and in particular of sexual relations with both female and male persons, be they free or slaves.
- *What I may see or hear in the course of the treatment* or even outside of the treatment in regard to the life of men, which on no account one must spread abroad, *I will keep to myself*, holding such things shameful to be spoken about.
- If I fulfil this oath and do not violate it, may it be granted to me to enjoy life and art, being honoured with fame among all men for all time to come; if I transgress it and swear falsely, may the opposite of all this be my lot.

(cited in Miles, 2005).

For medical professionals, abiding by the principle of non-maleficence as outlined in the Hippocratic Oath was challenged by the activities involving medical professionals in World War II. Experiments conducted by Dr Josef Mengele in Nazi Europe and by physicians attached to the Japanese military galvanised the world. The initial phase of the post-war Nuremberg Trials was conducted from November 1945 to October 1946. These trials aimed to prosecute prominent members of the political, military and economic leadership of Nazi Germany in the immediate period following the war. Subsequent trials ensued, including from December 1946 to August 1947, which resulted in the prosecution of 20 medical doctors involved in experimentation upon prisoners and the extermination of millions of persons in concentration camps and hospitals during the war. The experiences of World War II also had a significant impact on the nursing profession. Kappeli (2007) argues that it was during this period that 'the final loss of innocence of a humanitarian profession under the conditions of a dictatorship occurred' (2007: 248). In 1939, a law for the regulation of the nursing profession was enacted in Germany, with nurses required to swear an oath of loyalty to the Führer of the German Reich. In this way, nurses became involved in all the measures of Nazi health policies, including euthanasia programs and experimentation on prisoners (Kappeli, 2007). Some nurses refused to participate in the implementation of some Nazi medical policies that led to the harm and death of patients in their care. Despite this, nurse academic Rebecca McFarland-Icke states that during World War II, German nurses 'made choices, and their choices added up to the betrayal of thousands of people who were utterly dependent on them' (1999: 13). Interestingly, scholarship about healthcare ethics and the role of nurses in activities of the Third Reich has increased over the last few decades, with a large focus on conscience, moral distress and coercion in decision-making. There has also been significant academic discussion on the question of whether this experience of nursing in Germany during the war has any relevance for nursing as a profession in the twenty-first century. Key areas of focus in this academic discussion relate to the role of nurses in Nazi euthanasia programs, as well as that of nurses in the area of palliative care, particularly in countries where assisted dying and euthanasia are legal.

Following the Nuremberg Trials, international human rights charters, health professional charters, codes of conduct and codes of ethics were developed. Each of these was created in response to the atrocities against human persons that occurred on all fronts during World War II – not just in Europe. In 1948, the Declaration of Geneva was adopted by the General Assembly of the World Medical Association. This has been labelled as the Hippocratic Oath 'Mark II': it is regarded as a modernisation of the ancient medical professional code that aimed to affirm a physician's dedication to the humanitarian goals of medicine. Three key statements in the Declaration of Geneva (World Medical Association, 1948) are:

- I solemnly pledge to consecrate my life to the service of humanity.
- The health of my patient will be my first consideration.
- I will not use my medical knowledge to violate human rights and civil liberties, even under threat.

Such a Declaration was deemed to be essential by the medical profession at this time, given the implicit involvement of doctors in the atrocities of World War II. At the same time as the Declaration of Geneva was being formulated, the United Nations (UN) was created with the purpose of developing an international community that vowed never to allow the atrocities that occurred during the war to occur again in human history. World leaders who formed part of this first General Assembly of the United Nations decided to develop a charter that guaranteed the rights of all human persons. In 1948, the United Nations General Assembly adopted The Universal Declaration of Human Rights (UDHR). The Preamble of the UDHR (United Nations General Assembly, 1948) states the following:

> Now, Therefore THE GENERAL ASSEMBLY proclaims THIS UNIVERSAL DECLARATION OF HUMAN RIGHTS as a common standard of achievement for all peoples and all nations, to the end that every individual and every organ of society, keeping this Declaration constantly in mind, shall strive by teaching and education to promote respect for these rights and freedoms and by progressive measures, national and international, to secure their universal and effective recognition and observance, both among the peoples of Member States themselves and among the peoples of territories under their jurisdiction.

As a founding member of the United Nations, Australia played a prominent role in drafting the Universal Declaration. The head of Australia's delegation to the United Nations was Dr H.V. Evatt, who became President of the UN General Assembly in 1948. In this same year, the UDHR was adopted. Ratification of the UDHR covenants has been made by the Australian Commonwealth Government, and our courts are encouraged to take into account the stated provisions of the Declaration. The Commonwealth Government has passed specific legislation that gives effect to many of the rights set down in international instruments such as the UDHR. These include:

- the *Australian Human Rights Commission Act 1986*
- the *Age Discrimination Act 2004*
- the *Disability Discrimination Act 1992*
- the *Race Discrimination Act 1975*
- the *Sex Discrimination Act 1984.*

The Australian Human Rights Commission (AHRC) administers these Acts, and is empowered by federal law to hear and conciliate complaints from individuals who believe their rights have been breached.

Following the UN General Assembly's adoption of the UDHR, the next most prominent international declaration that had direct ties to the wartime atrocities was the Declaration of Helsinki, which was codified at the 1964 World Medical Association Congress. This new Declaration had the purpose of being a 'statement of ethical principles for medical research involving human subjects, including research on identifiable human material and data'. Again, the involvement of health professionals in the unethical and murderous experimentation on human persons in the name of science during World War II was at the forefront of the Declaration of Helsinki. This Declaration has become the foundation of many ethical codes of conduct and legal frameworks regulating research of human subjects, including the Australian National Health and Medical Research Council's (NHMRC) National Statement on Ethical Conduct in Human Research, implemented nationally in 2007.

Ethics in the context of the twenty-first century

To set the scene for this chapter and this book, it is helpful to consider how we live today and how we think about the way we live today. A number of circumstances that have shaped our society are pertinent here. The 1960s was a time of discovery of the joy of living, having moved on from the tragedy of the experience of a world at war in the 1940s and the literal rebuilding of social and economic life in Western society. The world – at least what was termed 'the Western world' – was reasonably prosperous; the shackles of the economic Depression of the 1930s and the legacy of two world wars had been shaken off and new movements abounded. Instead of embracing material prosperity, to some extent we embraced love, generosity and altruism. We decided that civil rights were important, that personal freedoms were worth defending, that the brotherhood of man (as it was described in those days) should become the solidarity of all people, although there was little acknowledgement that substantial changes like feminism – or at least the equality of women – were here to stay. People embraced technological change, and medical advances were (and remain) hugely popular; the space race captured our imaginations; the environmental movement began. Probably two of the most significant social changes that occurred at this time were the development of effective, cheap, reliable female-focused contraception and, linked to this, the desire/need for women to pursue careers of their own.

It is worth reflecting on our reactions to many of these joyous initiatives. We still have the contraceptive pill, but the 1960s dream of unfettered free love came up against AIDS and sexually transmitted diseases; the *freedom* for women to continue working after marriage and particularly after having children has become an *obligation* for them to do so. It is with some irony that those with significant disposable resources – 'the rich' – choose to return to work quickly, while those with very limited resources and little ability to find flexible employment – 'the poor' – are coerced into returning to poorly paid employment. Medical advances mean that it is frequently possible to keep people alive long after their brain has ceased to function – or, indeed, in the absence of a brain at all! Today the burning question is less about the preservation of life and more about how long we should keep going – and, more controversially, whether as a society we should allow or encourage or demand that people in certain health conditions should have their lives intentionally ended. Healthcare professionals are increasingly required to assess overall health needs and become community care assessors rather than being able to focus on their own areas of clinical and professional expertise. Career aspirations within most professions mean that you need to develop quite different skill sets: to advance very far in nursing, teaching or social work, you need to be good with budgets. Each division of an enterprise has a devolved budget, and one of the markers of your success as a manager, coordinator or team leader is the balancing of that budget. Finding new ways to limit expenditure or generate income is simply expected. It is one of the pragmatic reasons for the development of inter-professional approaches to healthcare and, while still in its infancy, to the development of inter-professional approaches to the *ethics* of healthcare.

Because of all these sets of circumstances, our ethical constructs, frameworks and guidelines are under significant stress. The guidelines, precepts and rules of the past may no longer seem relevant – or, at least, are in a situation where they are open to major questioning. In other words, as you read this you are thinking about it and assessing it in quite different ways than might have been the case for your parents or grandparents at your age and point in their careers. These illustrations highlight why the subject-matter of ethics is interesting, and why it should be of interest to you. Professionally, it is vital that you take the time to think and learn as much as you can because you will need to know and understand what you think and why you think it in order to best serve your patients/clients and your profession. As you read the various sections of this book, you should try to retain in the forefront of your mind two questions: What do you *really think* about the issues raised in the book? And *why* do you think what you do?

Studying 'professional ethics'

When an occupation has been determined to be one of the 'professions', it is considered to have a body of specialist knowledge obtained through substantial study, a set of required applied skills organised around that knowledge and a developed sense of ethics or ethical standards that guide the members of the profession in their practice of professional knowledge and skills. As Freegard (2007: 94) indicates, 'The standards to which members of a profession are to hold themselves are usually expressed in a professional code of ethics or conduct, which is promulgated and enforced by their professional association'. Such codes of conduct and ethics are normative frameworks to guide health professionals' moral conduct in their day-to-day clinical practice. Many professional bodies have position statements that form the basis of the collective affirmation of ethical conduct required of members within their profession in situations of moral uncertainty in practice. Of interest, prominent Australian healthcare ethicists Kerridge, Lowe and Stewart (2009) argue that the modern emphasis on professionalism in healthcare has gone too far. They state:

> Professionalism centres on the practitioner, and discussions about the professionalism seem sometimes to even ignore the existence of the patient. It is important for all health professionals to bear in mind that patient autonomy, patients' rights and patients' needs and desires are key ... not the autonomy, rights and interests of the profession. (2009: 120)

However, it could be argued that normative frameworks such as professional codes of ethics form the basis of the moral, social and professional values that are foundational and particular to members of that profession. They also provide evidence to society of the call for health professionals to protect and promote the welfare of persons in their care, and to avoid any self-interest that may pose a threat of harm or risk to the patient or client. They also affirm that the patient–health professional relationship is not just a service provision one typical of a free-market approach to consumerism. Health professionals bring to their daily role values, experience and knowledge that are not just prescriptive of a charter, code of conduct or ethical positions statement or code. The reciprocal nature of care between health professional and patient/client does not ignore the health professional's own rights in service provision and clinical practice. Most professional codes of ethics for health professionals, nationally and internationally, acknowledge this reciprocation and relationality between patient, their family, the community and the health professional. Therefore, such normative ethical frameworks for health professionals provide an orientation to the health professional and the general community with regard to expected behaviour and conduct in the provision of healthcare.

Professional codes of ethics for health professionals have evolved from international declarations and charters made following World War II. The 3rd General Assembly of the World Medical Association, held in London in October 1949, adopted the first Code of Medical Ethics that outlined the duties of physicians to patients, society and their profession. The International Council of Nurses first adapted a Code of Ethics for the nursing profession in 1953. This Code has been reviewed and revised several times since, with the most recent version being in 2012. The first Australian Code of Ethics for Nurses was developed and implemented in 1993 under the auspices of the Australian Nursing Council, the Royal College of Nursing, Australia and the Australian Nursing Federation. The most recent version of the Code of Ethics for Nurses and Midwives practising in Australia was released in 2008. In each of these Codes, eight value statements affirm the profession's commitment to respect, promote, protect and uphold the fundamental rights of people who are both the recipients and providers of nursing and midwifery healthcare in Australia. Speech Pathology Australia has also developed a Code of Ethics (2010) that aims to highlight the fundamental professional responsibilities of speech pathologists, and to affirm the highest standards of integrity and ethical practice. The Australian Association of Occupational Therapists' National Code of Ethics (2001) is founded on the principles of beneficence, non-maleficence, honesty, veracity, confidentiality, justice, respect and autonomy. Currently in Australia, the health professional groups of paramedicine and physiotherapy do not have professional codes of ethics statements.

These professional codes of ethics form the basis for fostering collaboration among members of health professional teams in the clinical setting. These codes have some common foundational values and principles; however, they also present variance based on scope of practice, professional regulation and accreditation. Traditionally, ethical reasoning in healthcare has been the domain of the medical profession, and usually focuses on the doctor–patient relationship. However, through the education of other health professions in ethical reasoning, the development of professional position statements on contentious issues in clinical practice, the implementation of professional codes of ethics and the involvement of nursing and allied health professionals in institutional healthcare ethics teams, ethical reasoning has become increasingly collaborative, and relies on an inter-professional approach. Interestingly, there is a lack of research on such collaboration between health professionals on ethical issues encountered in practice. Clark, Cott and Drinka (2007) argue that inter-professional moral reasoning is essential, due to the expanding scope of practice for health professionals in the clinical setting. They state that:

> The field of interprofessional education and practice is beginning to recognise the need for greater conceptual clarity and theoretical sophistication, so it is an opportune time to develop a comprehensive framework that will help to delineate issues and chart areas for further exploration in interprofessional ethics. (2007: 601)

As a healthcare organisation develops, and the numbers of health professional services and therefore teams also increase, the moral obligation of the providers of care from a professional and institutional context also needs to be recognised and developed. Inter-professional ethics, as an emerging field of professional discourse, is essential to respond to the changing needs of healthcare service delivery, and the increasing involvement of professional groups other than the traditional medical model in the deliberation on ethical issues in healthcare.

Bioethics or the ethics of healthcare?

As previously highlighted, the specific discipline of bioethics was one of the legacies of World War II. Because of the context that gave rise to this area of study the focus has tended to be very specific: largely focused on the situations of people in Western countries, and often just focused on specific issues such as end of life care, reproductive technologies, transplantation, resource allocation and experimentation. The responses developed have varied in their approach, but there have been three dominant forms of reasoning that have been applied to bioethics.

The most pervasive of these has been what has been termed the 'principles' approach, which is exemplified in the work of James Childress and Thomas Beauchamp (2012). These scholars identified four key principles:

- respect for autonomy – people should consent to treatments and to being party to research
- non-maleficence – healthcare professionals should always avoid harming patients/clients
- beneficence – healthcare professionals should always seek to benefit their patients/clients
- justice – resources should be allocated fairly within a healthcare system.

This approach has informed most professional codes of ethics. It is a form of prescriptive ethics – no action can be legitimate if it violates one of the principles. One of the key strengths of a principles approach has been the ease with which people can remember the terms – autonomy, non-maleficence, beneficence, justice – and then apply them. One of the key issues is that those terms are very context driven, meaning that they are not easily applicable in cultural or social contexts other than a Western construct. For example, the principle of beneficence – to do good – is not the same in a war zone as it is in a major metropolitan area in peacetime; nor is healthcare delivery in a desperately poor nation the same as it is in a wealthy nation.

Another major approach is utilitarianism. This approach to philosophy, and more particularly to ethics, derives from the philosophers Jeremy Bentham (1748–1832) and John Stuart Mill (1806–73). In its purest form, it holds that one should always act to maximise the good. What 'the good' might be is construed differently by different people: for some, it is hedonistic or equated with pleasure; for others, it is about happiness – which is more complex than just pleasure. Happiness can be very sophisticated – the joy of achievement, of seeing one's legacy carried on by children, leading a successful life and so on. Utilitarianism is a consequential theory – that the merit or goodness of an action can only be determined from its consequences. A significant strength of this kind of model is that it argues for maximising the good for the most people – it sounds democratic. Its most significant flaw is that only those whose voices are loudest or whose lives are not detrimental to the good actually count – hence the 'majority' whose happiness is maximised is the majority of those who count, and this almost always excludes minorities or those who exist at the margins of society, whose lives can be regarded as not conducive to the good. In terms of healthcare, this approach has been used to argue that there should be restrictions on access to healthcare resources for the elderly, people who live with disability and those who suffer from chronic illness. In some societies, it is also used to discriminate against children, the unborn, women and people of diverse gender and sexual orientation. Only the views of those deemed to be the majority count.

A third model is termed teleological, which means to examine the end-point or ultimate goal of an activity (or form of existence), and to ask whether or not a particular decision or action is in accord with the ultimate goal of the activity, existence or being. This type of ethical theory derives from the writings of Plato and Aristotle in ancient Greece, Anselm and Aquinas in medieval Europe and, in more modern times, Elizabeth Anscombe and Philippa Foot. It holds that all choices made and actions conducted should be in accord with the ultimate end or purpose of each human being, rather than the maximal good or happiness of the majority of people. It relies on understanding what things are (nature) and their end or purpose (*telos*). In this way, it can be understood to be holistic – as needing to consider the whole of the moral context and the person, as well as the particular instance before making a decision. In this sense, it requires knowledge of the who, the what, the how and the why. It is more challenging and complex than other ethical theories, and takes time – it is not a helpful approach if one is looking for a quick answer. A strength of this approach is that it does take time, and asks that a decision-maker consider many sides to an issue. It does not prefer a particular outcome or course of action; rather, it seeks to promote the well-being of the person and, in this particular context, the goals of healthcare itself. Given the increasing interest in inter-professional approaches to healthcare and the ethics of healthcare, this approach might have more to offer than other models precisely because it seeks to ask the professional to consider a variety of viewpoints before reaching an ethical decision.

Why study healthcare ethics?

This brief chapter has tried to set the scene for the rest of the book by setting out some of the reasons for studying healthcare ethics – it is a field of immense interest for anyone, but of deep and abiding interest for those who work in the field. The various healthcare professions require their members to adhere to codes of ethics; to really do this, the professional not only needs to know the code but also to understand where it came from and the models of reasoning that have been used in developing it, so that the professional can reason and apply the principles and codes.

The dedication required to graduate and maintain professionalism as a physiotherapist, speech pathologist, nurse, occupational therapist, midwife, paramedic or physician demands competence, knowledge and skill. It also demands a willingness to engage with the big questions of life, especially the questions of how we should live and die. Thus being a healthcare professional in the contemporary world also means being competent, knowledgeable and skilled in the field of healthcare ethics.

Reflective exercises

1.1 Map out a historical timeframe for the development of international charters or codes that health professionals may apply as a guide for moral conduct in healthcare.

1.2 Possessing a professional code of ethics is viewed as an essential element of professionalism. What implications does NOT having such a code have for health practitioners and professionalism?

1.3 Ethical reasoning in the healthcare domain is essential to the practice of healthcare professionals. Discuss and provide reasons for your answer.

1.4 Would there be a value in developing a universal Code of Professional Ethics for all healthcare professionals that presents an inter-professional response to ethical issues in the healthcare context? Discuss.

1.5 What are the similarities and differences in the ethical theories outlined above?

References

Australian Association of Occupational Therapists. (2001). *Code of ethics*. Retrieved 20 August 2014 from <http://www.otaus.com.au>.

Beauchamp, T. L. & Childress, J. F. (2012). *Principles of biomedical ethics* (7th ed.). Oxford: Oxford University Press.

Clark, P. G., Cott, C. & Drinka, T. J. (2007). Theory and practice in interprofessional ethics: A framework for understanding ethical issues in health care teams. *Journal of Interprofessional Care*. 21(6): 591–603.

Freegard, H. (ed). (2007). *Ethical practice for health professionals*. Melbourne: Cengage.

Kappeli, S. (2007). Reawakening memory: The Nuremberg congress – medicine and conscience 50 years after the Nuremberg trial of German doctors. *Medicine, Conflict and Survival*, 13(3): 245–53.

Kerridge, I., Lowe, M. & Stewart, C. (2009). *Ethics and law for the health professions*. Sydney: Federation Press

Klein, S. (1989). Platonic virtue theory and business ethics. *Business & Professional Ethics Journal*, 8(4): 522–3.

McFarland-Icke, R. (1999). *Nurses in Nazi Germany: Moral choice in history*. Princeton, NJ: Princeton University Press.

Miles, S. H. (2005). *The Hippocratic Oath and the ethics of medicine*. Oxford: Oxford University Press.

Nursing and Midwifery Board of Australia (2008a). Code of Ethics for Midwives in Australia. Retrieved 14 August 2014 from <http://www.nursingmidwiferyboard.gov.au>.

—— (2008b). Code of Ethics for Nurses in Australia. Retrieved 14 August 2014 from <http://www.nursingmidwiferyboard.gov.au>.

Speech Pathology Australia (2010). *Code of ethics*. Melbourne: Speech Pathology Association of Australia.

United Nations General Assembly (1948). The Universal Declaration of Human Rights. Retrieved 20 May 2014 from <http://www.un.org/en/documents/udhr>.

World Medical Association (1948). *Declaration of Geneva*. Retrieved 20 May 2014 from <http://www.wma.net>.

—— (1964). *Declaration of Helsinki*. Retrieved 20 May 2014 from <http://www.wma.net>.

2 Ethical theories

Jānis (John) Ozoliņš

This chapter begins with the question 'What is ethics?' It is not just a list of prohibitions, but rather a reflection on what we consider to be good or bad. It involves an evaluative and disciplined study of what we regard as morally good and what we see as morally bad. This is required if we are to decide how to act. Moral judgements, it will be shown in this chapter, are not simply based on what we think, but on ethical theories. There are two kinds of ethical theories: meta-ethical theories and normative ethical theories. The former are about the kinds of ways in which we can think about the nature of ethical principles and judgements, such as whether they are conventional or universal. Normative ethical theories provide a framework of moral principles that can help us decide whether or not an action is morally right.

Introduction: What is ethics?

Ethics, as it is commonly understood, is connected with various bans against wrong-doing – particularly in business or in the professions. In people's private lives, it is seen as demanding that, as far as possible, the actions someone chooses to perform have minimal effect on others around them – in some sense, that what people do is morally right. According to such a view, ethics is a means of regulating human behaviour, and so acts as a constraint on human action. This is, in fact, a very simplistic understanding of ethics. Ethics is not about any of the following:

- prohibitions concerned with sex
- ideal systems, such as codes of behaviour, which are all very noble in theory, but no good in practice
- something intelligible only in the context of religion, or
- personal likes and dislikes.

In other words, it is neither relative to a particular time, culture or place, nor is it merely the expression of subjective wants and desires (Singer, 2011).

Ethics is not just about sexual behaviour

From a meta-ethical perspective, ethics is about what we think is valuable and worthwhile to do as human beings, but it is sometimes wrongly thought that the main reason for ethics is to prevent people from indulging in sexual activity that is proscribed. That is, ethics is mostly concerned with the regulation of sexual activity between people. Despite the lurid obsession in the tabloid press with the sexual (and other) activities of celebrities, it is only one element of ethics, and certainly not its main preoccupation. It is true, for example, that such sexual activities as sex with children and coercive sex such as rape are universally regarded as morally wrong, as are sexual abuse and exploitation of others, but this is in the context of ethical values and beliefs about what is right and wrong. Various other related kinds of sexual activities involving violence, coercion and the inflicting of degrading acts on others are also condemned as morally wrong because of a particular set of moral values. It is this that determines whether certain sexual activities are morally wrong. For many in Western society, for example, various other sexual activities – provided that they do not harm anyone – are not regarded as morally wrong. Many people regard premarital sex between two consenting adults as not morally wrong. On some sexual matters, it is evident that there is no uniform view, so it is perhaps understandable that where there is a difference of view, those who hold that premarital sex is morally permissible will feel constrained if they live in a community where it is condemned. That this is the case, however, does not mean that ethics reduces to the prohibition of sexual activity.

There are therefore two ways in which the idea that ethics is about the regulation of sexual behaviour can be regarded. First, in a permissive Western world, ethics appears to have a marginal role in the regulation of sexual behaviour because it is clear that, apart from sexual abuse, and degrading and coercive sexual acts, nothing else is condemned. If this is so, we can conclude that it is not particularly concerned with prohibitions about sex. Second, ethics is not solely concerned with prohibitions relating to sex, but about the ordering of relations between people. In relation to the first point, if sexual activity between people is a private matter, and provided no one is harmed, it can be indulged in without being regarded as morally wrong, then the claim that ethics is about prohibition of sexual activity is false. Sexual activity can include all manner of sexual acts, such as genital sex, oral sex, sado-masochistic sex, anal sex and masturbation, as well as variations on these. Since none of these acts is prohibited when done in private between consenting partners, ethics does not appear to be specifically about sexual matters. It is important to consider that the term 'prohibited' may be deemed ambiguous because, in some countries, certain sexual activities are banned by law; in most Western countries, this is not the case. However, we can take prohibited to mean proscribed by some ethical beliefs and values. It is not the sexual acts themselves that are condemned, but the harm done to the partner whose trust has been betrayed. This suggests that ethics is not about prohibitions but, at the very least, about those acts that persons commit that do no harm to others.

It is useful to reflect on the reasons why it is claimed that ethics is not about prohibitions to do with sex. Even when we consider the views of those who hold that ethics is not needed to regulate what consenting adults do in private, the salient point is that it is not needed because the sexual activity occurs between consenting adults. That is, it is between individuals who are in some kind of consensual relationship with each other. It is presumed that what individuals choose to do in privacy is not an ethical matter because it is entirely their business. Whether or not this is the case requires further discussion, but its justification rests on the assumption that individuals are free to regulate their relationships with one another as they choose, with the proviso that no one is harmed. The moral rightness or wrongness hinges on whether an act causes harm to someone. Ethics is not about prohibiting acts as much as it is about prohibiting harm from being done to human beings as a result of the acts or omissions of others. Moreover, it is also clear that since harm can arise from acts and omissions, in some form ethics is about the relationships between people and the values and beliefs that regulate our actions.

Ethics is not about codes of behaviour

Second, ethics is not about ideal systems – such as codes of behaviour – that are aspirational, and that no one is really expected to live up to. This means ethics is not simply a list of general principles that set out rules of behaviour or conduct that are unattainable or so abstract that they are of no practical use in guiding actual behaviour. Thus a promise to be faithful to one's spouse can be held to be aspirational, but is practically impossible to achieve, since human experience tells us that the philandering husband and faithless wife are not rarities. General ethical principles are important, since they provide practical guidelines for ethical decision-making. For example, the Golden Rule – 'Do to others only what you would want them to do to you' – is general by itself, but leads us to ask how this broad principle can be implemented in actual ethical decision-making. That is, we can readily appreciate that the rule prohibits us from stealing and lying to others, since we would not want people to steal or lie to us. More positively, we would want people to keep promises they had made to us, and so we should – if we follow the Golden Rule – keep promises to them. The examples show that the Golden Rule has a practical application once we begin to think of actual situations in which it applies. What is morally good will be what accords with the Golden Rule, and what is morally bad will be what does not.

Codes of behaviour, however, do not guarantee that individuals will act according to the guidelines for behaviour that have been provided. This is perhaps the origin of the claim that codes of behaviour are of no practical use in daily life, since they only express ideals that no one can possibly meet. Ethics is much more than just a code of behaviour, because a code acts as a guide, not as a prescription for each and every act of moral decision-making. The claim that codes of behaviour are of no practical use in guiding actual behaviour is too strong, since even as a general principle the Golden Rule can direct our actions in a certain direction. Since codes of behaviour provide elaborated guiding principles for moral decision-making and action, we can expect that they will provide better guidance on how to act. Despite this, however, not every situation will enable the straightforward application of a guiding principle. Individual situations are unique, and will require application of a general principle to a particular case. It may not always be obvious how to apply a general principle to a particular case, and principles may also clash. For example, a hospital administrator may realise that the policy of decreasing the length of hospital stays will free up beds, but it may also result in an increase in the number of discharged patients who develop complications as a result of early discharge, as the resources to support them at home are lacking. Here two principles – distributing scarce resources efficiently and effectively, and providing the healthcare that individuals need – clash. This demands that ethical agents have not only knowledge of codes of behaviour, but also an understanding of what it means to act ethically. Codes of ethics are guidelines but, like all guidelines, demand an understanding of the moral principles on which they are founded, and how they can be applied in a given situation. The moral sense, in other words, is not captured simply by attempting to adhere to a code of behaviour. This does not mean that codes of behaviour are impractical, but that their application demands a degree of practical wisdom.

Ethics is not about religion

The claim that ethics is intelligible only in the context of religion is clearly false, since it is obvious that the obligation to treat others with respect and to act according to the Golden Rule is a universal requirement, and not simply one that is peculiar to religious individuals. Neither is it the case that ethics is justified only in terms of religious belief. There are a number of ethical theories that do not depend for their justification on religion or religious belief. Consequentialism, virtue ethics and deontology, for example, do not depend on religious belief for their justification. In contrast, religion and religious belief are not solely concerned with the regulation of moral behaviour and the prohibition of what a particular religion regards as immoral acts. There is a popular view, reinforced by the media, that religious leaders of all faiths seem to be concerned with enforcing a particular moral code that regulates human behaviour. It can be admitted that there is some foundation for this view, since both ethics and religion are concerned with the relationships among human beings and, in religion's case, the relationships between human beings and God. Importantly, religions call human beings to follow a particular kind of life, and ethical behaviour towards others will be a significant living out of the religious life. This adds an extra dimension to the understanding of the imperative to treat others with respect, and to only do to them what we would want them to do to us.

The major religions of the world – Buddhism, Christianity, Hinduism and Islam – all provide a religious context in which ethical behaviour is not only a part of practising the particular religion but also the context within which it is justified. Buddhism, for example, enjoins its adherents to seek nirvana – a state of moral and spiritual perfection – through living their lives in accordance with Buddhist teachings. Although Buddhism does not subscribe to a supreme being, its teachings are to be understood as guiding principles in the living of a life aimed at virtuousness, which is to say a life aimed at moral perfection and fulfilment for oneself and for others. Similarly, Hinduism is based on sacred writings – the *Vedas* – that consist of myths, stories and rituals for sacrifices. These writings provide a guiding framework for the ordering of a moral life. Practising Hindus are called upon to find their place within a hierarchy, not only of fellow human beings but also of the natural world of plants and animals, as well as within the cosmos. To act morally is to act in accordance with one's place in the cosmos. Dharma, a key concept in Hinduism, represents both conformity of the individual to the standards of behaviour required by their position in society and the totality of the norms required by every individual in every caste in order to maintain cosmic order. It is evident from these two examples that, for believers, religion provides a context for ethical behaviour – and, it can be added, for the normative ethical theories that provide the principles guiding moral decision-making and action. It is important to note that, for non-believers, there is little or no acceptance of metaphysical presuppositions that underlie religious morality. Religion, however, is not just about moral behaviour, but rather about an understanding of the place of the human being in the world, and their individual relationship to it. For monotheistic religions such as Christianity, Judaism and Islam, it is also about the relationship between human beings and God.

The claim that ethics is only intelligible in the context of religion is based on the observation that religions provide a system of beliefs about the universe, its origins and the place of human beings within it, as well as a comprehensive system of values that order the relationships human beings have with each other and with what transcends human existence. In the case of Buddhism, human existence is directed to reaching nirvana, a transcendent state of freedom from suffering. Unlike monotheistic religions, the Buddhist conception of transcendence does not imply or require the existence of God. The upshot of this is that an atheist, who does not believe in a personal God or any kind of Supreme Being but is prepared to accept some kind of transcendent reality, could accept Buddhist ethics. Moreover, taking this one step further, the atheist could adopt some of the ethical principles of Buddhism without subscribing to its view of transcendence, replacing this with a general conception of contributing to the good of humanity through ethical behaviour. Thus an atheist who does not accept any kind of transcendent reality could nevertheless accept the general ethical principles that have their foundation in Buddhism. Clearly, some other metaphysical justification for adopting these principles would be required, but there is no logical reason why this would not be possible. Alternatively, the non-religious believer could simply ignore the need for a justification of moral principles and claim that they are self-evident. From this we can conclude that, although it is true that ethics is intelligible in the context of religion, this is not its only context.

This conclusion is further strengthened by the observation that Aristotle (1976), in developing his theory of virtue ethics, relies not on religion but rather on an understanding of what is good for human beings. By carefully examining various candidates for what could be considered good for human beings, Aristotle concludes that the answer is not fame, fortune or power, but virtue.

Similarly, in developing the foundations of moral action, Kant (1998) proposes the hallmark of morally right action is acting in conformity with a good will, which means being willing to act in conformity with what is a rationally morally good action – that is, one that rationally agrees with what is demanded by a universal maxim. Religion does not play a part in Kant's deontological theory.

Ethics is not just a private matter

A common view is that the ethical principles held by individuals are entirely a private matter. This view is often invoked in the public arena, where it is argued that no one should be allowed to impose their views on another. The justification for such a view is generally made on the grounds that autonomous human beings have a right to decide the values by which they will live their lives, and others have an obligation to allow them to do so without interference or constraint. Leaving aside the question of the extent to which individuals are entitled to autonomous choice of values and to act on these within a society with a plurality of beliefs and values, there is a conflating of two separate issues within the aforementioned justification. The first issue concerns the extent to which human beings are able to be autonomous within a community of equals, a question addressed by Hobbes (1991), by whose bleak view human beings could not be trusted to learn to get along with each other and make allowances for different wants and desires, but needed to be ruled by someone – Leviathan – who could impose right order on unruly citizens. Although individuals can be completely autonomous in their decision-making, in that they can decide what they want to do, they may not be able to act because they might be prevented from doing so by others. The second issue concerns the extent to which ethical values are a matter of subjective decision. In other words, the extent to which what is morally right or wrong is decided by how an agent feels at a particular time and in a specific situation. If autonomy is absolute, no one has a right to question the specific moral values held by a person. The question is the old one that Plato (1987) argued about with Protagoras, namely whether 'man is the measure of all things'. Plato did not think the human person was the measure of all things. It is this second issue that most often leads to the view that individual subjective views about moral matters are private and beyond criticism.

Some simple examples illustrate how the view that ethical values are subjective is untenable. Suppose a well-known medical researcher asks her research assistant to alter some data so that it supports a particular theoretical position, but undermines that of a rival with whom she is competing for much-needed funds. These funds include a component from which the research assistant's salary is paid. It goes without saying that the assistant is dependent on the income that is received from his job. If ethics is subjective – that is, if we act according to self-interest – then self-interest dictates that he will alter the data (after all, no one will find out . . . he hopes) and the medical researcher for whom he works will receive the funds to keep him in employment. Since self-interest is the determining factor, his actions are morally right, given that what is ethical depends only on his subjective preferences at that time. However, the next day he receives a job offer from his boss's rival, and he decides to refuse to change the data. His action is again morally right, since self-interest determines what is ethical, but crucially it makes his action the previous day morally wrong, since he is now of the view that he should not change the data. Two different actions – one the opposite of the other – are morally right depending on an individual's subjective assessment at a particular time. It should also be noted that if moral values are subjective, then the research assistant's colleague, who thinks that it is morally wrong to falsify data under any circumstances, is also right in her judgement. This is an absurd situation, but perhaps the position can be saved.

Leaving aside objections that the research assistant is relatively powerless, and so his decision-making is to some extent compelled, it could be objected that he acts consistently with his own self-interest in both cases. It is not unreasonable that he should want to keep his job. This can be conceded, but the central question is whether self-interest is a suitable principle to serve as a determinant of what is morally right or wrong, and so ethical decision-making. In order to be able to consider this, we need to define what we mean by self-interest. We can define self-interest as that which we subjectively regard as being good for us as individuals, and what is good for us is the achievement of our wants and desires. If ethics is subjective, then acting in such a way that we achieve what we regard as our good, whatever that may be since we define it, is morally good. This will also mean that any means we choose to achieve our wants and desires will also unquestionably be morally good, since they serve our self-interest, which is our guiding moral principle.

Unfortunately, self-interest fails as a guiding moral principle. It fails because wants and desires fluctuate, and so do our judgements about what is to our personal advantage. What someone desires on one day may be different to what they may desire on another day. As we saw above, conflicting self-interested situations lead to different ethical positions. It is also the case that individuals who seek to gratify their desires become enslaved by them.

Self-interest dictates that they act in accordance with them because the good is defined in terms of the achievement of the wants and desires that individuals have. Hence someone driven by the desire for wealth will become a slave to their passion. Self-interested persons have no interest in anyone or any thing that does not further their own interests, and so their horizons extend no further than themselves and their world shrinks to a narrow preoccupation with themselves. They are moved to engage with others only insofar as it enables them to get what they want. They become incapable of authentic relationships with others, since because they are driven by self-interest, their only reason for fostering a relationship is to further their own objectives. A single-minded pursuit of individual wants and desires, however, relies upon other human beings, since the achievement of fame, fortune or power is not possible without others. This means that because they are incapable of relationships with others for their own sake, they will use other persons as means, reducing them to objects, indistinguishable from other kinds of objects. Their world lacks a human dimension, and they have become almost inhuman themselves. Self-interest therefore cannot serve as the guiding moral principle if the aim of ethics is human flourishing. This means that we cannot be subjective about ethics.

Meta-ethics and normative ethics

Ethics can be divided into three parts: meta-ethics, normative ethics and applied ethics. The last of these, as the name suggests, deals with ethical theory applied in particular contexts. Here we will concern ourselves with the first two, since we need to have some understanding of ethical theories and their content in order to be able to apply ethical principles in applied contexts. Meta-ethics is about ethics in general; it is about the genesis of ethical theories and the basis of our ethical reasoning. Ethics itself is about what is good – that is, what makes some actions good rather than bad. In fact, some of our previous discussion has been engaging in meta-ethics. Asking whether self-interest is sufficient as a guiding principle for ethics is a meta-ethical question. Some of the questions asked by meta-ethics, therefore, are about the nature of moral goodness: about what makes something right or wrong, whether moral propositions can be true or false and whether there can be universal ethical theories or whether they are restricted to a particular time, culture and tradition. There are a number of different meta-ethical theories, and these provide particular approaches to our understanding of ethics. We will now briefly discuss some of the main meta-ethical theories.

Meta-ethical theories

Meta-ethical theories – or, more precisely, approaches to ethics – can be divided along two axes. On one side of the first axis we have theories that espouse moral realism; and on the other side, we have theories that promote moral anti-realism. Along the other axis, orthogonal to the first, we can divide approaches to ethics between cognitivist accounts and non-cognitivist accounts. Classification of the various meta-ethical theories is not an exact science, and some theories will overlap the axes, but it is useful to have a general understanding of the range of meta-ethical theories, their differences and their similarities. The four quadrants are moral realist and cognitivist; moral realist and non-cognitivist; moral anti-realist and cognitivist; and moral anti-realist and non-cognitivist.

- *Moral realism* is the view that when we make statements such as 'Lying is wrong', and 'One should keep one's promises', these are capable of being true or false. Moreover, moral realists also believe that not only are some such statements capable of being true or false, but some of these statements actually *are* true and can be shown to be true. Moral facts, in other words, are true whether we agree with them or not. Moral realism claims that moral facts are mind independent.

- *Moral anti-realism* rejects the idea that there are moral facts, so that when we make moral statements, we are not making statements that are capable of being true or false. This means that in making moral statements or making moral judgements, we are not basing them on moral facts, so they are not true or false in the same way that non-moral statements are. Moral anti-realists do not deny that we sometimes speak as if there are moral facts, but they argue that these are human constructions that regulate our relationships with others. Hence 'You should keep your promises' is true not because of some objective features of the world, but because human beings, through experience of relationships with one another, have constructed a way of understanding and negotiating those relationships so that it is true that promise-keeping is right. Anti-realists therefore deny any independent moral realm in the world, arguing that morality is a construction of human minds.

- *Cognitivism*, in general, is the claim that a proposition, such as 'The ball is red' can be either true or false, describing an actual state of affairs in the world. It is therefore possible to test the truth claims of the proposition that 'The ball is red' against a feature of the world. Moral cognitivism is the view that moral claims are about moral facts about the world, and so will be either true or false. Cognitivism requires an account of the nature of knowledge, since the claim is that there are facts about the world that we can know which are independent of how we might think about them. Hence, if 'Lying is wrong' is a moral fact, then we need to be able to show how we come to know that this is true.

- *Non-cognitivists* deny that moral claims are about what can be demonstrated as an objective fact about the world – that is, they deny that moral statements are capable of being true or false. Instead, the moral non-cognitivist holds that moral claims express preferences about desires, feelings and attitudes. Moral claims and judgements are ways of expressing how we feel about a situation, and do not state facts about the world. Non-cognitivism allows that we might prescribe certain kinds of behaviour in certain situations; however, this has nothing to do with moral facts, but is rather an expression of common feelings that people have about certain actions. Lying is wrong because it makes us feel bad, for example.

Most moral realists will also be cognitivists, since they think that it can be demonstrated that some moral statements are actually true. In the same way, a statement in the moral sphere, such as 'Lying is wrong', points to an objective feature of the world, and can be established by pointing to a feature of the world. Anti-realist cognitivists would hold that statements in the moral sphere can be about what is true or false; however, this is not about features of the world, but rather about the moral domain that human beings have constructed. If there is a moral fact about the world, it will be so because human beings have created it as a means of constructing relationships with one another and regulating them. They can, however, be cognitivist, since they can accept that within the construction of morality there can be moral statements that are true or false, but that these are not about the world; they are about a socially fabricated subjective human construct.

The anti-realist non-cognitivist, like the anti-realist cognitivist, believes that morality is a socially fabricated construct, but denies that there are any statements made within that construct that are either true or false. At best, in this case, moral statements will be conventions, agreed to by human beings. Hume (1998) argues that morality is an expression of likes and dislikes, and because human beings are very similar to one another, it is not surprising that they will have the same likes and dislikes. What disgusts one person is very likely to disgust another, and what one person likes is very probably going to be something that is liked by another. Morality in this case largely reduces to a matter of taste – though for Hume there will be some commonalities in what human beings find good and pleasurable.

There are many different meta-ethical theories, and they will fit the four classifications that we have outlined to different degrees, as there is always some argument about whether a theory is cognitivist or non-cognitivist, as well as about the extent to which it is realist or anti-realist. We briefly discuss some examples of theories that fall within each of the classifications, bearing in mind that there are variations among all of them. Debates between different proponents of various meta-ethical theories have dominated discussion of moral philosophy for centuries, and anti-realists' claims that the lack of agreement about the basic concepts of morality point to its lack of reality, and that it is really about desires and preferences, have some justification.

Moral theories that fall into the moral realist and cognitivist category will have their foundation in some form of naturalism, which claims that there are certain features of what it is to be a human being that dictate our ways of acting towards others. Natural law theory, for instance, is a moral realist and cognitivist theory, since it claims that there is a distinct human nature, and that by examining the features of human experience, it is possible to determine what is good for human beings. What is good for human beings is not a matter for conjecture, but is an objective feature of the natural world. The truth of statements such as 'Killing of innocent human beings is wrong' can be established by reference to the basic human goods, one of which is the good of life. Another theory that falls into this category is virtue ethics, which also claims that it is possible to specify what constitutes the good for human beings. For the virtue ethicist, human flourishing or human fulfilment is obtained through the practice of virtue. What is good is what leads to virtue, and virtue leads to the ultimate end of human beings, which is happiness.

In the moral realist and non-cognitivist category are those moral realists who agree that there are some moral statements that are true or false, but as a matter of fact, it is not possible to establish *which* are true or false. It follows that we deny that there are ordinary means to establish the truth or falsity of moral statements. Error theorists, such as J. L. Mackie (1977), hold that it is the case that some moral statements are true or false, but as a matter of fact it is not possible to establish these as such. What this means is that, although there is agreement that there are moral statements that are true or false, there is no agreement about which statements are which. Consequentialism, for example, holds in its simplest form that an action is good if, on balance, it is better to act in one way rather than another. Put another way, an act is good if it leads to the greatest good for the greatest number. Here we can agree that some statements can be true or false, but which ones are true can never be determined ahead of assessing a particular situation.

In the anti-realist and cognitivist category, the claim is that our moral theories are a human construction, and so do not appeal to an independent metaphysical reality. Anti-realism is generally taken to imply a form of idealism, which is to say that whatever it is that we know about the world it is mind-dependent. In its classical formulation, idealism claims that all we can know about the world is our perception of it and, more strongly, that the world is just perception. Moral anti-realism therefore holds that moral theory is constructed from our experiences, which shape our accounts of what is morally right and morally good, independently of an objective reality. That is, what is morally right and good will depend in some way on normative judgements about how rational agents will act in certain circumstances. Kantian ethics is usually thought to fall into the anti-realist and cognitivist camp, although it is true that some Kantians defend a realist interpretation of Kantian ethics. Arguably, Kant (1998) can be defended as an anti-realist because he holds that we cannot know the *noumenon* – the thing-in-itself – but only the phenomenon – how it acts on us – although it is to be acknowledged that this is far from a decisive argument in relation to Kantian ethics.

In the fourth category, the anti-realist and anti-cognitivist quadrant, theories deny that there are any moral statements that are true or false, from which it also follows that they deny that we are capable of knowing any moral statements that are true or false. It also follows that there are no means for establishing the truth or falsity of moral statements. Various subjectivist theories fall into this category, including expressivism, emotivism and intuitivism. Expressivism, for example, claims that moral statements are expressions of particular preferences. Moral statements are descriptions of what moral agents hold about particular actions and situations without holding that what is described refers to an objective state of affairs. Thus, if we claim that torture of children is wrong, this is because we are expressing a particular attitude towards torture of children. We do not like it, or we are disgusted by it. On the other hand, if we say that we like bondage and sado-masochism, we are expressing our liking for it, and hence it is not morally wrong but morally right. A moral theory that falls into this category denies that there is an objective moral realm.

As is apparent, there is a great diversity of views about the nature of the good, about what is morally right or wrong and whether the truth or falsity of moral judgements can be established. Informing these questions are differing conceptions of human nature, the relationships between persons and the ultimate end of human beings. Different understandings of these will, to a great extent, determine our moral commitments. From the diversity of meta-ethical theories emerge a number of normative ethical theories that assume that concepts such as the good, positive and negative freedom, moral rightness and wrongness are understood. Most normative ethical theories agree on the need for the principles of moral decision-making to be universal. That is, the moral principles that guide our decision-making need to be able to be applied consistently and rationally in a variety of contexts and circumstances. This does not mean that there will not be differences of opinion among people about what is thought to be morally right, even when they apply the same set of normative moral principles to the same case. Differences will be the result of different perspectives of the state of affairs on which a moral judgement is going to be made, and the variety of assessments possible that can be made of a particular situation.

Normative ethics and ethical theories

Normative ethics is concerned with what makes some actions morally good rather than morally bad, and how we decide this. It is therefore concerned with theories about what is morally good and what is morally bad in terms of action or what agents do. Unlike meta-ethics, however, normative ethics is not concerned so much with the nature of moral goodness, but about establishing guiding principles to help decide whether an action is morally good or bad. It is therefore the disciplined, rational study of moral judgements, and of how to make them by applying a consistent set of moral principles. This is important if we want to be able to make consistently good moral decisions; otherwise it is highly likely that our decision-making will be haphazard and inconsistent. Normative theories also claim to be universal – that is, a crucial feature is that they go beyond individual likes and preferences. While it is not expected that everyone will adopt the same normative ethical theory, they will at least be able to recognise the universal applicability of the theory. Significantly, as the term 'normative' suggests, normative ethical theories seek to establish moral principles that most people would regard as having some binding force, which is to say that they are rules that most people would regard as establishing clearly what is morally right and what is morally wrong. Hence, for example, while not everyone subscribes to a religious basis for their normative moral principles, they certainly recognise the universal nature of the moral principles that are embodied in the Ten Commandments. These provide normative rules that are considered binding on everyone, not just believers. This means that 'it is wrong to take innocent life' is a moral rule binding on everyone. Different normative ethical theories will have different ways of establishing the moral principles and rules that are claimed to be binding on everyone.

Some of the most common normative ethical theories are utilitarianism (a species of consequentialism), deontological theories, virtue ethics and natural law. These will be further discussed individually in separate chapters. We will provide a brief outline of them below.

Utilitarianism

There are many varieties of utilitarianism, which is a form of consequentialism because an important feature of every variety of utilitarianism is that it seeks to weigh up the good that comes from pursuing a particular course of action as opposed to another. This will mean that the utilitarian will take into account the consequences of a decision to act in a particular way. As the name suggests, utilitarianism assesses the utility of a particular course of action as opposed to another, weighing up whether it is better to do one thing rather than another. The morally good act will be the one that produces the greatest amount of good. Classical utilitarianism, such as the views held by John Stuart Mill (2009) and Jeremy Bentham (1907), identified the good with pleasure, so the act that is to be chosen will be one that produces the greatest amount of pleasure. Even though Mill offers a sophisticated account of pleasure, other utilitarians are mindful of the criticisms that are made of his account, and develop other versions of utilitarianism. Utilitarianism is a universal moral theory because it provides a way of weighing up courses of action according to normative rules that can be applied by anyone, and so is not reliant on the subjective likes and dislikes of any individual.

Deontological moral theories

Deontological moral theories can be contrasted with consequentialist theories in that they do not begin with a consideration of whether one act results in better consequences than another, but on whether it is right to act in a particular way. For the deontologist, it is not a matter of determining whether an act brings about more good, but whether it is the right thing to do. There is a duty or obligation to do what is right, even if it does not lead to the greater overall good. For example, if it is wrong to steal, then even if by stealing a loaf of bread an agent could prevent someone from starving to death, it would be wrong to do so. More starkly, although a consequentialist might accept the idea that an innocent life could be sacrificed for the greater good, a deontologist would not, since the duty or obligation to preserve life is what matters, not whether an action leads to good consequences. What is important for the deontologist is that we do what is right, and that means that we take the obligations and duties we have to others as determining whether the action we perform is morally right, and so good because it is right. Deontology is also a universal normative ethical theory, since it claims that our duties and obligations are determined by a rational consideration of our relationships with others and what we owe them.

Natural law theory

Natural law theory can be construed broadly as the view that human nature is such that in order for human beings to flourish and to lead lives that lead them to the good, they are bound by natural law. This law can be construed to be a divine law, ordained by God, that is inscribed in the minds of all human beings. The natural law theory emphasises the importance of the good, since natural laws outline how human beings are to act in order to do what is good, which directs them to their final end: God. Natural law says that there are universal basic human goods that all human beings need in order to lead happy and fulfilled lives. The most basic human good is the good of life. Natural law theorists hold that a careful study of human nature will reveal the basic human goods that all human beings need in order for them to live. Natural law theory is a universal normative theory because it holds that all human beings need the basic goods in order to live and to flourish, and from these basic goods it is possible to develop moral principles that act as guidelines to moral decision-making and moral action, which is good.

Virtue ethics

The fourth major normative ethical theory is called virtue ethics. In Western philosophy, it is usually Aristotle's (1976) account of virtue ethics in the *Nichomachean Ethics* that is its most influential source. In Eastern philosophy, its major counterpart is classical Confucian ethics. Virtue ethics concentrates first on considering what is good for human beings; having reflected on this, Aristotle concludes that what is good for human beings is virtue. Virtue itself, however, is in need of explanation, and Aristotle explains that virtue is connected with doing that which leads to human fulfilment, and the ultimate end of human life is happiness. Practice of the virtues therefore leads to human fulfilment and happiness. In virtue ethics, to act in a morally right way is to act in accordance with a particular moral virtue. The moral virtuous person is not someone who acts morally well in a particular situation, but someone who strives to act morally well in *every* situation. That is, they develop a habit of acting well, and hence develop a particular virtue. For example, in order to be temperate – which is to say possess the virtue of temperance – it is not enough to act once or twice in a temperate fashion; it needs to be a part of a person's essential make-up. What is morally good will be determined by whether an act contributes to the develop-ment of virtue, and hence leads persons to their good, which is happiness. Virtue ethics is a universal normative ethical theory because it holds that the same virtues are required by all human beings if they are to flourish and to also obtain happiness.

Conclusion

In this chapter, we have looked first at the nature of ethics. It was argued that it is much more than just prohibitions about sex, and that it is not merely about codes of ethics or based on religion. Nor is ethics about personal likes and dislikes. Ethics can be understood to have three divisions: meta-ethics, norma-tive ethics and applied ethics. Applied ethics, which deals with the application of normative ethical theory in specific contexts, was put aside to outline the distinctions between meta-ethics and normative ethics. In meta-ethics, impor-tant questions are raised about the nature of moral good, and whether it can be known. Depending on our answers to these questions, normative ethical the-ories could be classified into four broad divisions: moral realism and cogniti-vism; moral realism and non-cognitivism; moral anti-realism and cognitivism; and moral anti-realism and anti-cognitivism. Some ethical theories could be said to fall neatly within one of these divisions, but others are not so easy to classify.

Four normative ethical theories were introduced: consequentialism, deon-tology, natural law and virtue ethics. Each of these has a particular way of understanding the nature of the good, and of what constitutes a morally good action. The consequentialist holds that it is a matter of being able to assess the consequences of a particular choice, the deontologist whether the action accords with what is right and with one's duty, the natural law theorist whether the action is in accordance with the basic human goods and the virtue ethicist whether the action leads to growth in virtue, and hence happiness.

We conclude with a few points that need to be taken into account in ethical decision-making:

- We should seek to understand the issue as fully as we can.
- We need to understand the context of the situation within which we are to make our ethical decision.
- We need to know what our moral values are, and be able to justify them.
- We need to be aware of the constraints and limits of our responsibility. It may not be within our competence to make a decision, and we may need to seek assistance.
- In contemplating an action, we should familiarise ourselves with every possible solution and consider how the solution we choose accords with our moral values. We should also be aware that there may not be a solution, and we may have to act as best we can.
- Whatever the situation, we should not only choose a good moral action, but also base our decisions on the importance of acting justly.

Reflective exercises

2.1 The introduction to this chapter presents a series of statements about what ethics 'is not', then discusses these in depth. Summarise each of these statements and reflect upon them in relation to your private and professional life.

2.2 What are the main differences between meta-ethics, normative ethics and applied ethics? Where does the study of healthcare ethics fit within these branches of ethics?

2.3 There is a great diversity of views about the nature of 'the good', and what is morally right and wrong. What are some of the cultural, legal, social, spiritual and relational elements that influence your understanding of 'the good' in both your private sphere and your clinical practice? Do you think there may be any occasions that present a dilemma between your understanding of 'the good', private or professionally?

2.4 Is there a difference between doing what is good and doing what is right?

2.5 Discuss the statement: 'I don't need to know any ethical theories to know how to act morally.' How would you justify such a statement?

2.6 Summarise the key components of each normative ethical theory presented in this chapter and, through additional self-directed learning, identify a key historical and a contemporary author in healthcare literature that supports these frameworks for ethical reasoning:

- utilitarianism
- deontological theories
- natural law
- virtue ethics.

References

Aristotle (1976). *Nichomachean ethics*, trans. J. A. K. Thomson, introduction and bibliography Jonathan Barnes (rev. ed. with notes and appendices H. Tredinnick). Harmondsworth: Penguin.

Bentham, J. (1907). *An introduction to the principles of morals and legislation*. Oxford: Clarendon Press.

Hobbes, T. (1991). *Leviathan*, ed. R. Tuck. Cambridge: Cambridge University Press.

Hume, D. (1998). *An enquiry concerning the principles of morals*, ed. T. L. Beauchamp, Oxford: Clarendon Press.

Kant, I. (1998). *Groundwork for the metaphysics of morals*, trans. and ed. Mary McGregor. Cambridge: Cambridge University Press.

Mackie, J. L. (1977) *Ethics: Inventing right and wrong*. Harmondsworth: Penguin.

Mill, J. S. (2009). *Utilitarianism*. (1879 ed.). Auckland: The Floating Press.

Plato (1987). *Theaetetus*, trans. and essay Robin A. H. Waterfield. Harmondsworth: Penguin.

Singer, P. (2011). *Practical ethics* (3rd ed.). Cambridge: Cambridge University Press.

3 Ethical principlism

Jānis (John) Ozoliņš

Ethical principlism is a popular ethical theory in healthcare ethics. It is based around four principles: beneficence, non-maleficence, autonomy and justice. Some codes of ethics, which try to provide guidance in healthcare, make use of these principles. This chapter will first explore what each of these principles involves, consider some examples of the principles in action and look at some of the difficulties and limitations of principlism. Principlism is at its best when the four principles work together to provide a framework for moral action, and at its worst when principles come into conflict. For example, showing respect for patient autonomy may not always lead to treatment that would be in a patient's best interests, and so could conflict with the principle of beneficence.

It is no surprise that when we discuss standards of moral conduct or seek guidance in moral decision-making that we appeal to moral principles that help us make decisions about how we should act. Different normative moral theories have different starting points, so we can arrive at different views about what is good and what is morally right. Different theories, starting from different principles, result in different moral rules.[1] This suggests that where there are challenging moral issues in the healthcare area, there will be considerable difficulty in finding agreement about what course of action is morally appropriate. Ethical principlism is a possible way forward: it proposes that, despite differences among ethical theories, there is a common core morality, and invites us to consider our moral decision-making within a framework of four moral principles. That is, it is claimed that whatever our starting point in moral theory might be – whether it is utilitarianism, virtue ethics, deontology or natural law – if we begin from the framework of ethical principlism, then the more likely we are to reach an agreed decision on a moral question. The appeal of ethical principlism is that it will help us to make justifiable moral decisions rather than establish what is objectively morally right. Principlism assumes that because there will be an overlap among the various moral rules enunciated by different normative theories which yield a common core morality, there will be acceptance of the four principles that form the framework within which moral questions are considered.

Ethical principlism is not entirely new, since the utilisation of moral principles in medical ethics was appreciated by John Gregory (1724–73), who wrote on medical ethics in response to the state of medicine in England in the eighteenth century. Gregory outlined an approach to the treatment of patients in response to what he saw as the chaos that was medical treatment in eighteenth-century England. More often than not, physicians would hold off treating patients if there was a likelihood that they might not respond to treatment, as a poor outcome would do damage to their reputations and thus their incomes. Gregory argued that sympathy and service were important principles in the care of patients (McCullough, 1996). More recently, the Belmont Report (National Commission for the Protection of Human Subjects of Biomedical and Behavioral Research, 1979) provided a brief outline of the ethical principles that should guide medical practice and research. Written in reaction to some extent to the revelations during the Nuremberg war crimes trials about the abuses of human beings in the conduct of medical experiments in Nazi Germany, the Belmont Report outlined the principles that should guide medical research, noting that the distinction between healthcare research and practice is not always clear-cut. Because it is experimental, a new treatment designed for the care of a particular patient could be considered research. The Belmont Report identified three basic principles in the Western tradition that it claimed provided a justification for many ethical prescriptions and evaluations of human actions: respect for persons, beneficence and justice. Drawing on the Belmont Report, Beauchamp and Childress (2013) have extended the basic principles to four by splitting beneficence and adding non-maleficence to the other three. They have been widely recognised as providing one of the most developed accounts of ethical principlism. In what follows, we will first consider what is meant by a principle, discuss the plausibility of a common morality as required by ethical principlism and provide an outline of each of the ethical principles.

What is a principle?

Though principles can be thought of as general guidelines for moral decision-making and moral rules as being more specific articulations of them, the term 'principle' has also been used interchangeably with the term 'rule'. Thus the term 'moral principles' has been used to describe the moral rules which form the basis of an ethical theory. Moral rules, which are constitutive of an ethical theory, provide the justification for choosing to act in one way rather than another, since they determine which acts, according to the rules applied, are morally good or bad. Thus, for a preference utilitarian, a basic principle is that we should maximise our preferences. In moral reasoning, judgements about how to act begin from a general principle that is applied in a specific case so that a conclusion is reached, which is then acted upon. R.M. Hare (1952: 56) uses the terms 'principle' and 'rule' interchangeably, noting that if someone decides not to tell a lie in a particular situation it is because they are acting according to a principle, such as, 'Never tell lies'. In general, it is not possible to make any value judgements without having some principles and/or rules that act as guides to action. This is because judgement involves an examination of the situation and its evaluation according to a set of principles. If we consider the question, 'How ought we to act?', it is clear that there is no specific answer unless we have some principles that will guide our actions. If we consider as an analogous question, 'How ought we to drive?', we cannot respond without some principles to guide our driving. Depending on the country, an important principle is to recognise that we drive on the left: it is not a matter of deciding on a different side each day. Driving rules enable every licensed driver to be able to drive on the road without creating chaos and accidents because no one is adhering to any rules or principles.

It is important to realise that principles that guide us in response to the question 'How ought we to act?' are not logical rules of inference, since the question also asks for a value judgement to be made in response to the assessment of a particular situation. For example, in a simple application of a rule of logic, such as *modus ponens*, the conclusion follows logically. Thus, in the following application of *modus ponens*, provided the first two statements are true, the conclusion will also be true: If this is a mule, then it is barren. This is a mule. Therefore it is barren. Ethical principles do not operate in this way, because in every case a value judgement enters the reasoning process. This means that there is always room for a different conclusion to be reached. For example, suppose our principle is, 'In Australia drive on the left.' A simple application of *modus ponens* gives us: If we are in Australia then we drive on the left. We are in Australia; therefore we drive on the left. This is straightforward. Now suppose the left-hand side of the road has crumbled and it is dangerous to drive on the left. Here we need to make a practical judgement about whether we adhere to the rule, since the over-arching reason for driving on the left is to drive safely because we value our safety and that of others. Driving rules are not merely logical rules of inference, but rather principles that act as guidelines to ensure the good of driver safety and the smooth flow of traffic. Similarly, ethical principles are guidelines that take into account what we value, and are not rules of inference that will allow us to determine a course of action merely by applying logical reasoning. For example, *modus ponens* gives us: If this is a lie, do not say it. This is a lie; therefore do not say it. Suppose you are treating a patient who is very ill with an uncertain prognosis, but who you have good reason to suspect will deteriorate very quickly if you were to inform her of her condition. If she asks you, 'Am I going to die?' it is not so obvious what the answer should be. Principles can only be guides; the hard work of making practical decisions still remains.

There are three reasons why we need principles. First, if we are to choose a particular course of action, we need to have some basis for making the choice, otherwise it is arbitrary. And while it is possible to act arbitrarily – just as it is possible to choose a different side of the road on which to drive each day – the resulting chaos is not desirable. Second, we need principles because they provide us with a consistent guide to how we should act, enable conformity with our values and bring orderliness to our decision-making. They also signpost what is the good for us. Third, without principles of some kind, it is not possible for someone to learn or be taught anything at all. This is because it is through principles and rules that we distil what we know so that we have guidelines for helping us to make decisions. These cannot be private principles, since – as we have already shown in relation to driving – we all need to drive on the same side of the road if we value our safety. Just as the rules of driving need to be taught, so too will ethical principles. If this is not done, the consequence is that the wisdom and values of a culture cannot be passed down to the next generation, since this is impossible without some ordering and classifying of knowledge (Hare, 1952).

To summarise, principles act as guidelines, since they are not simply rules of inference in the way that logical rules such as *modus ponens* are. It is also clear that they involve value judgements, and one principle may well clash with another, making decision-making complex. Valuing one principle more than another will lead to different decisions about courses of action. Principles can be considered standards or norms of conduct on which our judgments and decisions about how to act depend, forming the basis of our moral reasoning and conduct. More specific rules can be formulated based on principles, but neither these rules, nor judgements making use of these rules, can be deduced from them (Beauchamp, 2007).

Common morality

In order for the four principles to be effective, a crucial element is that there is some common understanding of morality. This makes sense, since – extending our driving analogy – it would be impossible to drive in other countries if road signs and road rules did not have some commonalities. We would be forced to learn new road rules each time we visited another country. Similarly, if we are to apply the four principles approach to moral issues, it would be very difficult, if not impossible, if there were no common moral principles. Beauchamp and Childress (2013), who have perhaps the best developed account of ethical principlism, argue that in every culture, there are core moral rules that are common to all cultures. That is, they claim that there are universal moral norms by which we can judge the actions of human beings. Some of these universal moral norms are familiar to us – for example, (1) do not kill; (2) do not cause suffering to others; (3) prevent evil or harm occurring; (4) rescue persons in danger; (5) tell the truth; (6) nurture the young and dependent; (7) keep your promises; (8) do not steal; (9) do not punish the innocent; and (10) obey just laws. In addition to these, they claim that there are moral standards or moral character traits other than these moral norms. There are at least 10 of these too: (1) non-malevolence; (2) honesty; (3) integrity; (4) conscientiousness; (5) trustworthiness; (6) fidelity; (7) gratitude; (8) truthfulness; (9) lovingness; and (10) kindness (2013: 3). These are not exhaustive, but indicate the range of moral norms and character traits that are claimed to be universally valued. On the other side of the coin, we recognise that certain other traits are not desirable, such as dishonesty, untrustworthiness, lack of concern for others and selfishness. These, too, are taken to be universally deplored. These universal moral norms and character traits are not divinely given, according to Beauchamp and Childress, but are the result of universal human experience and history. Moreover, it is claimed that their existence can be confirmed or disconfirmed by empirical scientific research.

The claim that there are common moral values is controversial, since it rests not only on asserting that there is a common human nature that is universally shared, but also on proposing that for the main part human beings are disposed to act virtuously. What is required is an anthropology that is able to explain why human beings seem to share various moral norms and character traits. The challenges for such an anthropology should not be underestimated, since many would argue that there is no common human nature because there is plenty of diversity among human beings (Trigg, 1988). A further complicating factor is that there is no consensus about how human nature is to be characterised. Some evolutionary biologists argue that common human nature is defined in terms of biology, and that what is essential about human beings is defined in terms of their DNA. Others point out that no two human beings – save for identical twins – share the same DNA, so there is debate about the extent to which we want to claim that human beings have a common biological nature (Pinker, 2002).

The problem of identifying the essential nature of human beings would not become any easier even if we were to ignore small differences in DNA and concentrate on the attributes that human beings share. Nor are we any better off using a more coarse-grained approach to conceiving of human nature, since evolutionary biology has shown that there are no fixed properties among organisms considered to be members of the same species (Dawkins, 1988). Nevertheless, this has not prevented evolutionary biologists from proposing more sophisticated biological explanations of human characteristics and behaviours that, it is claimed, capture the essence of what it is to be a human being. The difficulty is that these discussions leave untouched questions about what is right and wrong, even if a 'criminal' gene were to be identified.

On the other hand, a conception of human nature that ignores the biologically embodied reality of human life, and attempts to characterise human nature in historical, cultural and social terms alone, is also misguided. Human nature is not merely a human construction that is culturally and historically bound, and so different at diverse times and places that there can be no common human nature. Human beings need to eat, drink, sleep, avoid pain and procreate, just like other animals, and this is not historically or culturally constructed. That they also seek the companionship of others, crave recognition and status, and organise themselves into groups, tribes and communities, can also be attributed to the kinds of biological creatures they are. For different peoples, human culture and history arise out of reflection on particular shared human experiences, and out of this comes a shared understanding of human nature that is expressed in literature, poetry and religion. It is because there is diversity in how these experiences are expressed that a variety of perspectives on human nature can be constructed. The plausibility of the claim that there is a common morality rests on being able to show that what arises from a diverse human experience is a consciousness that human beings, through the exercise of free will, are able to choose actions that lead to their flourishing.

An understanding of the nature of human beings is crucial to deciding who is to be considered to have moral status and who does not. Typically, we accord lesser moral status to non-human animals. The four principles are not normally applied to them. The question of to whom the four principles are to be applied, however, becomes fraught when we consider human beings, and to whom among them we apply the four principles. For example, the moral status of human embryos, human foetuses, children, the disabled, and the frail and elderly will depend on whether they satisfy the conception of human nature that is chosen by those who have the responsibility for looking after their interests.

Although we do not intend discussing moral status here, it is important to be aware of its effect on how and to whom ethical principles will apply. We will take the view that they should apply to all human beings from conception, since a new human individual, whole and entire, comes into existence on the completion of syngamy. A human embryo is a human being at the earliest stage of development, but possesses all the epigenetic primordia that is required to reach adulthood via self-directed means. Including all human beings and excluding none means that we include those with genetic defects, those with disabilities, those with dementia and brain damage, those in a state of post-coma unresponsiveness, the very young, the very old and those who are unable to exercise any of their capacities as human beings. A broad definition of moral status ensures that no one is excluded from consideration in the application of ethical principles because they may lack certain capacities, and ensures they are admitted to membership of the moral community. This is important because, in those cases where human beings have a diminished capacity to exercise their own decision-making powers, members of the community are obliged to do so on their behalf.

We will not consider whether some non-human animals, such as the great apes, have moral status. It may be the case that moral status applies more broadly than just to human beings. Discussion of this question will take us deeper into an account of moral status than we wish to go here. Pinker (2002), for example, argues that there is neuro-scientific and behavioural evidence that supports his view that there is a universal human nature that is biologically based. For the present, we will confine ourselves to a consideration of the ethical principles as they apply to human beings, as we have defined them.

The four principles

Autonomy

Respect for the autonomy of the individual person is one of the key principles of modern bioethics. In the Western liberal tradition, personal autonomy is the capacity to act freely in making decisions in accordance with choices that have been determined by the individual, acting without interference from others. In making choices, individuals do so with understanding and by making full use of their critical mental capacities, such as reasoning ability and intentionality. The two most important characteristics of the autonomous person are the ability to be able to freely and independently make decisions and the ability to exercise judgement. To respect autonomous agents is to affirm their right to exercise their right to independently make choices and act according to their principles, values and beliefs, without coercion from others (Beauchamp et al., 2008). It is evident that respect for autonomy takes place within a community of other human beings.

There are several theories of autonomy. Some concentrate on the capacities of individuals to be self-governing – that is, being able to reason, understand, manage and deliberate – while others focus on the ability to make choices, distinguishing between first-order preferences or desires, and higher level second-order preferences. First-order preferences typically are associated with basic needs or desires, such as for food, drink and sex, whereas second-order preferences are associated with longer term and higher goals, such as the desire for health, for good relationships and success in a career. In some cases, basic desires will clash with second-order preferences, and where persons give in to basic desires, they are not acting autonomously. For example, an alcoholic may realise that, for the sake of his health, he should not drink, so he has a higher level preference to preserve his health. If he chooses not to drink, he is acting on his higher level preference, and so acting autonomously. On the other hand, if the lower order preference – the desire for alcohol – is overwhelmingly strong and he succumbs, then he is not acting autonomously (Beauchamp & Childress, 2013). A difficulty with such split-level theories of autonomy is that a very strong basic or first-level preference can determine a second-order preference. For example, someone overcome with desire for another's spouse may develop a plan to initiate an adulterous relationship. Here, the extent to which an individual is truly acting autonomously becomes questionable.

An alternative to split-level theories of autonomy is the three-condition theory, in which autonomous action is understood in terms of normal choosers who act (1) intentionally, (2) with understanding and (3) without controlling influences that determine their actions (Beauchamp & Childress, 2013: 104–5). Intentional actions are those where agents deliberate about the actions they plan to take and volitionally carry them out. Intentional actions can be a series of separate actions that are designed to reach a particular goal, or they can be just one action that agents plan on doing. Intentional actions will be actions that agents purposefully and consciously seek to carry out. For example, a patient may have a goal of returning to health, and so will carefully undertake all those actions prescribed by her healthcare team. For instance, she can take her prescribed tablets each day, or she will exercise for 30 minutes daily and eat healthy food. Each of these actions is undertaken intentionally, since the patient intends to attain a long-term goal. Each of the individual actions themselves is also intentionally undertaken, since the agent does them purposively and deliberately. In contrast, non-intentional actions are those that are side-effects of an intentional action or accidental. For example, in raising an arm to wave to a friend, a person may unintentionally bump someone standing next them. The bump was unintended, but raising the arm in order to wave to a friend was intended.

The second condition, understanding, requires agents to understand what it is that they are choosing. Agents who do not understand what they are choosing to do are not acting autonomously, since they do not know what they are doing. There are two ways in which understanding may be lacking: (1) the agent does not understand what actions need to be carried out in order to achieve a particular desired result; and (2) the agent does not understand how to carry out the actions that are required to achieve the desired goal. In the first case, the agent may want to regain physical fitness and strength, but does not understand that this will require not just exercise, but regular aerobic and anaerobic exercise. In the second case, the agent may have been given a list of exercises to perform, but does not understand the instructions for how to do them properly. Full understanding is not necessary for autonomous action, since this is too strong a requirement, given that in most instances agents will not act with complete knowledge and understanding. The requirement is that agents have sufficient understanding to know what it is that they are knowingly choosing to do. The consequence of this is that agents are rarely able to act fully autonomously. This means that autonomy exists on a continuum, where some actions are fully autonomous, while others will be partly autonomous.

The third condition is that agents are able to act without controlling influences that determine how they act. That is, they are not constrained by either external conditions or by internal conditions that impede their ability to act. External conditions are of a variety of kinds. For example, an agent may wish to improve physical fitness by jogging for 30 minutes each day, but because of a large fall of snow, this is not possible. Here the external condition prevents the agent from acting. Internal conditions are also constraining on agents. For example, the agent may suffer from agoraphobia and so, if the aim is to become physically fit through jogging, then this will not be possible if the agent is prevented by his condition from stepping outside.

Though acts are either intentional or non-intentional, it is apparent that the second and third conditions offered for autonomy admit degrees. That is, it is possible to not have full understanding, but still to be able to exercise limited autonomy. In many cases, agents will not be certain that they have fully understood what steps are needed in order to achieve a particular goal, and to that extent will be not entirely in control. This will be the case particularly in issues to do with healthcare treatment. Agents will accept the advice of their healthcare practitioners, even while not fully understanding the proposed treatments. The decision to undergo the treatments is autonomous to the degree that the agents are able to understand how they will contribute to the regaining of their health.

Similarly, it is possible to be constrained by external and internal conditions to some extent without being prevented from exercising some autonomy. External conditions could be such things as pressure being placed on patients to undergo certain kinds of medical treatments – either by families who are anxious to see them recover, or by physicians and healthcare professionals who believe that they know what is in the best interests of patients. The level of pressure applied can be very variable. At one end of scale, patients cannot exercise any control over their treatment, while at the other end, they have complete autonomy. Internal conditions likewise can also reduce autonomy, since individuals who have some form of mental illness or some disability that affects their capacity to make decisions will be prevented from exercising autonomy fully.

Beneficence

Beneficence is the central goal of healthcare, since the care of patients is the reason for its existence. Beneficence involves not just treating persons with respect in their decision-making, but also in protecting them from harm and attempting to secure their well-being (National Commission for the Protection of Human Subjects of Biomedical and Behavioral Research, 1979). Beneficence has two imperatives: (1) do no harm; and (2) maximise possible benefits and minimise possible harms. The principle, 'First do no harm', or *primum non nocere*, is popularly ascribed to the Hippocratic Oath, but in fact does not appear in it in that form. It does, however, contain a promise that the physician will do no injury to their patients (Herrell, 2000). This principle, 'do no harm', is called the principle of non-maleficence, and is treated as a principle in its own right. The second imperative of beneficence can further be elaborated into three separate clauses of its own: (1) evil or harm ought to be prevented; (2) evil or harm ought to be removed; and (3) good ought to be done and promoted (Frankena, 1973). As can be seen, the first half of beneficence, or non-maleficence, deals with the imperative not to do harm, and so is a passive form of beneficence, since it does not enjoin healthcare practitioners to act, but rather to refrain from acting. The second imperative is active beneficence, since it requires action on the part of agents.

The three clauses elaborating active beneficence need further specification in order to provide practical guidance to action. In general, we understand beneficence to involve being kind to others, helping them, being generous to them, defending and protecting their rights, and being forgiving to them. These are positive actions that seem to apply to the third very general clause to promote and to do good. Preventing evil or harm to others could include rescuing them from danger, coming to their aid when they are in need and alerting them to the dangers of smoking, enacting legislation to improve road safety and initiating awareness of the importance of healthy eating. Removing evil or harm in some ways will overlap with some preventative measure, but in the healthcare area we can readily see that surgery to remove a cancerous growth is an obvious example of removal of an evil. It can also be seen as preventative, since it may prevent the proliferation of the cancer. (It is important to note that evil is being used in the sense of what is inimical to the well-being of human beings and not moral evil – that is, we are speaking of natural evils. An earthquake, for instance, is a natural evil, as is disease.)

Preventing and removing harms or evils is central to healthcare. Healthcare practitioners have a primary responsibility for the alleviation of suffering, and for the prevention and removal of harms. Curing of diseases, the binding of wounds, designing prosthetics, and researching and developing new drugs are all positive aspects of beneficence. In engaging in all these activities, healthcare practitioners need to be mindful of the risks involved in what they might propose in order to alleviate suffering and to prevent harms. For example, although a particular procedure will relieve a particular condition, it may be dangerous and, if unsuccessful, could leave a patient worse off than before. Treatment of an abscess on the spinal cord, for instance, may require its drainage, and there is the possibility of neurological damage that may result in paraplegia. While this is unlikely with modern treatment, nevertheless the treating healthcare professional needs to be aware of all the risks.

Beneficence does not oblige anyone to take extraordinary measures in order to prevent or remove evil and harms. For example, no one is obliged to donate a kidney in order to save another person. While altruism is to be admired, preventing harm to another does not require that an individual should inflict harm on their own person. In some other instances, there will be conflicting actions to be considered, and so limitations to the application of the principle of beneficence. A psychiatrist who learns that her client intends to murder someone will have an obligation to inform the relevant authorities in order that the murder be prevented. By informing the police, however, the psychiatrist is violating patient confidentiality, and thus undermining the relationship of trust that is crucial to being able to treat someone. If it became known that psychiatrists regularly provided information to the authorities about their clients, it is unlikely that they would be trusted again (Beauchamp & Childress, 2013). This example highlights that ethical principlism as a normative moral framework for health has *prima facie* limitations for healthcare professionals when applying these principles to a practice context.

Non-maleficence

The principle of non-maleficence emphasises that the treating healthcare professional will act in such a way as to cause no harm. It is evident that not causing harm is distinct from positive beneficial actions, which promote welfare, provide benefits and protect interests. Non-maleficence includes harms that are avoided, such as stealing from someone, and not causing disability or death. In the healthcare situation, non-maleficence does not mean that we avoid all harms, since it is sometimes necessary to cause harm in order for a greater good to be realised. For example, someone may be particularly sensitive to pain, but in order to effect a cure, some pain necessarily has to be inflicted. It is well known that certain cancer treatments such as chemotherapy and radiotherapy have significant side-effects that cause harm to the patient.

Nevertheless, in this instance, it is evident that undergoing treatment provides the best chance of survival.

Despite this, it is held that the principle of non-maleficence will, in a number of instances, take precedence over the principle of beneficence. For example, suppose a government decrees that prisoners on death row are to provide their organs for donation to those who are in grave need of transplants. A prisoner could therefore be required to donate various organs, such kidneys, heart and liver, because he could thereby save the lives of four people. In this case, if he had a choice, a prisoner would be acting reasonably if he refused to give his permission for the dividing up of his organs, even if such an action would bring about significant benefits to others. The principle of non-maleficence on this occasion overrules the harvesting of the prisoner's body for spare parts (Beauchamp & Childress, 2013).

Given that the principle of non-maleficence is defined negatively as 'do no harm', it is worth making some remarks about what is understood by harm. Harm can be understood in two ways: (1) X harms Y means that X wrongs Y – that is, X does something that violates a moral principle, for example, by lying or betraying Y's trust; and (2) X harms Y means that X afflicts Y – that is, X does something that thwarts, defeats or sets back Y's normal interests and goals. In the former case, X stands for the actions of another person, whereas in the second case, X can also stand for such things as natural disasters, disease and bad luck. It can also stand for something that a person has done, to which the second party consents. For example, a physician who amputates a limb does not do so without good reason. Loss of a limb is a harm, but if removal of it is done with the aim of saving the individual, then it is a justified harm. The principle of non-maleficence requires us to provide justification for any harm that we might cause.

Justice

Our encounter with justice usually begins from a very early age, when someone has taken a toy from us or refused to share their lollies with us. Our response is to cry that it is not fair, and to express our deep felt sense of injustice at the wrong that has been done to us. From an early age, we are aware of justice and conscious that wrongs have to be righted. The literature on the concept of justice is vast, and there are several different ways in which we can think about it. Our first encounters with justice alert us to retributive justice – the sense that wrongs have to be redressed – and to distributive justice – the sense that we have to be treated fairly in respect of what we receive. Other ways of thinking about justice include justice as what one deserves, whereby justice is understood as what we have merited and deserved. An additional way is for justice to be viewed as restorative justice, where restitution is made for what has been wrongfully damaged or destroyed, and social justice, which concerns itself with the common good. Each of these concerns itself with different aspects of justice, although there will be some commonalities. Retributive justice, for instance, contains the thought that it is fair to punish those who do wrong. In healthcare, we are mainly concerned with distributive justice, which involves justice as fairness.

Distributive justice is concerned with the distribution of social burdens, benefits and opportunities in a fair manner, so that one group in society does not bear the burdens of providing benefits while sharing in few of them, or receive more benefits than others in the community. Opportunities for education, health, welfare and jobs should also be equally shared, so that no one group in the community is excluded. Ensuring an equal distribution of healthcare is not as simple as the principle enunciated makes it sound. Even if we accept the formal principle of justice found in Aristotle's *Nichomachean Ethics* (2004) – namely, that equals should be treated as equals and unequals should be treated as unequals – the application of this principle is complex. This is because the principle does not specify what sense of equal is to be applied. Intuitively, we would suppose that it means that where two people have the same need, they will be treated in the same way. This is particularly important in healthcare, since there are scarce resources, and healthcare practitioners (as well as governments) are placed in the unenviable position of deciding how resources are to be distributed.

Following is an example of the difficulties of determining how to apply the formal principle of justice in a particular case. Suppose we have two individuals presenting at the emergency department of a busy hospital. One has a very bad cut and is bleeding profusely, while the other is complaining of feeling dizzy and having trouble standing up. Both require attention, but only one can be seen by the busy emergency department. The two individuals are equals in the sense that they both have equal moral status, but they are not equals in terms of who should be treated first. The second part of the principle could be invoked by providing reasons why they are unequal. It would make sense that the team would attend to the person bleeding profusely first, but this is by no means obvious. To help us decide, besides the formal principle of justice, we also need material principles, which specify the substantive conditions for fair distribution of resources, goods or services. These are sometimes called substantive principles of justice – that is, the practical principles that we need in order to apply the formal principle of justice. In addition to these, we can also appeal to procedural principles of justice – that is, the rules or procedures which we apply in order to do what is just or fair (Rawls, 1999). It is clear that the first material or substantive principle involves distribution according to need. Thus justice requires that each receives according to their need. In the case of healthcare resources, we would define a need as something that a person requires in order to avoid being harmed in some way. Hence the person bleeding profusely needs our attention first, since it is possible he could bleed to death if left unattended. This is an example of triage, a set of procedures that are employed in emergency departments in order to attend to patients according to need.

The following list of material principles provides some illustration of the kinds of principles that do or might form the basis of distributive justice:

- To each person an equal share.
- To each person according to individual need.
- To each person according to capacity for acquisition in the free market.
- To each person according to individual effort.
- To each person according to societal expectation.
- To each person according to their merit.

It is possible to accept all of the principles or only one or two, as well as to consider adding others to the six (Beauchamp et al., 2008: 26). It makes sense to use the material conditions that are most relevant in deciding what is just and fair. For healthcare, the first two material conditions will be most important. Applications of these conditions to particular cases are challenging, and different theories of justice have been developed that elaborate the material principles.

One such theory has been developed by John Rawls (1999), who proposes that we begin from a position in which persons constituting a society are free and equal. In such a society, the principles of justice will be those that free and rational persons would accept as furthering their own interests from an initial position of equality. Moreover, for a society in which all are to be treated justly, there has to be consensus about what these principles that constitute justice are. In order to determine principles that all can agree to accept, consensus is arrived at from behind a hypothetical 'veil of ignorance', in which no one in the decision-making process is aware of their position in society, wealth, status, intellect and so on. This is to ensure that no one will bias the principles to favour them personally. Rawls also proposes that any decisions about the principles of justice should ensure that the least fortunate in society are favoured.

The application of the principles of justice to healthcare is complex, and different situations make it difficult to rely on guidelines to provide solutions to the dilemmas faced by healthcare professionals. Although a theory of justice can help determine what a just level of patient care would be like, in the face of decisions about costs and resources, it cannot take the place of decision-making about how to choose to use those resources in particular circumstances. This will always remain a matter for deliberation and decision in individual cases (Buchanan, 2009).

Conclusion

Ethical principlism has the virtue of attempting to provide some principles for decision-making, particularly in terms of healthcare ethics that can be universally accepted. They point us to important general principles that need to be taken into consideration in the assessment of the treatment of patients. By themselves, however, they will not determine whether an action chosen will be morally right or wrong, since they rely on the details of what is morally right or wrong to be filled out by moral theory. A problem for ethical principlism is whether the principles as enunciated are sufficiently elaborated to provide genuine guidance in the difficult ethical situations that can arise in the healthcare context. Respect for the autonomy of the patient, for example, is important to acknowledge, but there may be occasions when the patient will not be well placed to make an autonomous decision. To justify over-riding a patient's autonomous choice will require justification, and this will require a moral theory that provides justification for the limitation of autonomy.

Reflective exercises

3.1 What is the difference between a principle, a rule, a law and a guide-line? What are some of the key factors influencing health professionals in appealing to ethical principles in ethical reasoning in clinical practice?

3.2 Beauchamp and Childress (2013) state that ethical principles are only *prima facie* in their application to moral deliberation. What does this mean, and what are the implications for ethical reasoning in clinical practice for the health professional, the patient and their family/next of kin?

3.3   Is paternalism ever ethically justifiable in the provision of healthcare? Discuss with relation to the care of vulnerable populations (e.g. children, the mentally ill and the elderly), and also in situations of clinical emergency.

3.4   Many modern medications, treatments or procedures have side-effects that may cause harm to the patients they benefit, with specific disease signs and symptoms. Does this mean that the principle of non-maleficence is always being violated?

3.5   Does the health professional have a duty of care to ensure that a patient's autonomous choice for provision of certain aspects of healthcare is fulfilled? Where do patient advocacy and conscientious objection fit within this reasoning?

3.6   Would it be ethically just for some members of the community to be denied access to treatment, given that their disease is caused by lifestyle choices, such as smoking, high-fat diets, a sedentary lifestyle and alcohol consumption?

Note

1.   We can distinguish principles, rules and norms, although the distinctions are not always clear-cut and these terms are sometimes used as if they were synonymous. Principles can be thought of as general precepts or postulates on which a moral theory is based. Hence, for example, a utilitarian would take 'the greatest good for the greatest number' as a general guiding principle. Rules would be a more specific articulation of the principles upon which the theory is based. Norms are also rules, but can be distinguished from rules by being rules that we are obliged or obligated to follow. Social norms, for example, are social behaviours to which we are expected to conform. Moral norms are the moral behaviours to which we are expected to conform. A moral rule, on the other hand, may be a specific requirement of a theory, but how it is understood in practice can be different, so a moral norm can be different from a moral rule. In natural law theory, moral norms are specific moral rules that everyone is expected to follow.

References

Aristotle (2004). *Nichomachean ethics*, trans and ed. Roger Crisp. Cambridge: Cambridge University Press.

Beauchamp, T.L. (2007). History and theory in 'applied ethics'. *Kennedy Institute Ethics Journal*, 17(1): 55–64.

Beauchamp, T.L. & Childress, J.F. (2013). *Principles of biomedical ethics* (7th ed.). New York: Oxford University Press.

Beauchamp, T.L., Walters, L., Kahn, J.P. & Mastroianni, A.C. (2008). *Contemporary issues in bioethics* (7th ed.). Belmont, CA: Thomson Wadsworth.

Buchanan, A. (2009). *Justice and health care: Selected essays*. Oxford: Oxford University Press.

Dawkins, R. (1988). *The blind watchmaker*. Harmondsworth: Penguin.

Frankena, W. (1973). *Ethics* (2nd ed.). Englewood Cliffs, NJ: Prentice Hall.

Hare, R.M. (1952). *The language of morals*. Oxford: Clarendon Press.

Herrell, H. (2000). *The Hippocratic Oath: A commentary and translation*. Retrieved 20 March 2014 from <http://utilis.net/hippo.htm>.

McCullough, L.B. (1996). Bioethics in the twenty-first century: Why we should pay attention to eighteenth-century medical ethics. *Kennedy Institute of Ethics Journal*, 6(4): 329–33

National Commission for the Protection of Human Subjects of Biomedical and Behavioral Research (1979). *The Belmont Report: Ethical principles and guidelines for the protection of human subjects of research*. Retrieved 20 March 2014 from <http://www.fda.gov>.

Pinker, S. (2002). *The blank slate: The modern denial of human nature*. New York: Viking.

Rawls, J. (1999). *A theory of justice*. Cambridge, MA: Belknap Press.

Trigg, R. (1988). *Ideas of human nature: An historical introduction*. Oxford: Basil Blackwell.

4 Personhood and human dignity

David G. Kirchhoffer

The concepts of personhood and human dignity are widely used in contemporary healthcare ethics. This chapter provides a brief overview of how the concept of human dignity came to be so important in healthcare ethics, and examines how the concept's widespread use and relationship to the concept of personhood have led to problems regarding its meaning and relevance. A practical solution is then presented.

The rise of the concept of human dignity in healthcare ethics

The word *dignity* is derived from the Latin *dignus*, which means worthy. Since dignity refers to worth, human dignity refers to the worth of the human. What makes the concept of human dignity important for ethics is that, unlike the dignity of a queen or the dignitaries at an awards ceremony, which expresses the worth or status of particular human individuals in relation to others, human dignity is meant to express a worth that is equally shared by all human individuals.[1] It is not meant to be dependent upon their social status, economic wealth, race, gender or anything else. Moreover, it is meant to affirm a worth beyond price. Human individuals are said to be moral goods or ends in themselves, not merely good or useful as means to achieving other ends.

The history of the concept of dignity goes back at least to ancient Greece and Rome. Cicero, for example, used dignity in both of the ways described above – that is, to refer to the special status of some people in the socio-political order (*De Inventione* 2.166) and to refer to the special status of all people in the natural order (*De Officiis* 1.106). The tension between these two understandings continues to the present day.

Human dignity and human rights

For healthcare ethics, probably the most important development in the use of the concept of human dignity is its inclusion in the United Nations' Universal Declaration of Human Rights (UN, 1948), hereafter referred to as the UDHR. During World War II, Nazi attempts to exterminate humans deemed inferior, and the Allied bombings of civilian populations in cities such as Dresden and Hiroshima, both displayed insufficient regard for the worth of human individuals. In the aftermath, there was a strong desire to ensure that this would never happen again. One way to do this was for all nations to affirm and protect by law the absolute worth of every human individual. Consequently, the 1945 UN Charter lists the reaffirmation of faith in 'the dignity and worth of the human person' among the primary aims of the UN. In 1948, this reaffirmation is further elaborated in the UDHR, which states in its preamble that 'recognition of the inherent dignity and of the equal and inalienable rights of all members of the human family is the foundation of freedom, justice and peace in the world'. In Article 1, the UDHR goes on to state that, 'All human beings are born free and equal in dignity and rights. They are endowed with reason and conscience and should act towards one another in a spirit of brotherhood.'

The high international standing of these documents meant that the concept of human dignity became firmly embedded in international human rights law. Because humans were recognised as having equal dignity or worth or moral status, they also all had equal rights – that is, entitlements to certain freedoms and to the provision of certain basic goods, such as food, education and so on, by the states of which they were citizens.

A brief survey of international human rights documents demonstrates an expanding awareness of the equal dignity of all human individuals. The UN produced binding international legislation to eliminate racial discrimination (1965), to secure civil, political, economic, cultural and social rights (UN, 1966a, 1966b), to eliminate discrimination against women (1979 – 31 years after the UDHR!), against cruel and inhuman punishment (1984), to secure the rights of children (1989), to protect the rights of migrant workers and their families (1990) and to protect the rights of people with disabilities (2006). Thus dignity and the rights that proceed from it are no longer the preserve of those who had historically held the power to decide who was worthy of moral concern – namely, upper-class European men.[2] Over the past 60 years, more and more people have been explicitly included as equals, and hence worthy of the same moral concern: people of colour, women, prisoners, children, migrants, people with disabilities and so on.

Not surprisingly, the concept of human dignity has also become important in healthcare ethics. There are power imbalances between healthcare
practitioners and patients, much as there were (and arguably still are) power
imbalances between those who were included in the circle of moral concern
prior to World War II and those who were excluded. These power imbalances
can have many facets. They may be physical (weak versus strong, ill versus
healthy), emotional (fearful versus confident), intellectual (ignorant versus
knowledgeable) or social (poor versus rich, male versus female). And the
practitioner is not always in the more powerful position. Two moral risks
arise from such power imbalances: first, there is a risk of losing sight of the
fundamental moral equality of patients and practitioners; and second, there is
a risk of treating patients differently based on their relative features – for
example, their race, gender, economic status, age or health. These risks are
heightened when decisions need to be made that will be detrimental for one of
the parties involved – such as in the allocation of limited resources or the
prioritisation of cases in an emergency room. What the concept of human
dignity does is affirm that all patients have a right to be treated with dignity,
in a manner that respects (is worthy of) their equal dignity or worth as human
individuals. Whatever decisions are made, and whatever actions are undertaken, should be made with due acknowledgement of this fundamental moral
equality.

Consequently, the UN's 2005 Universal Declaration on Bioethics and
Human Rights strongly emphasises human dignity, both as an aim of the
declaration and as one of the key principles to be applied in making ethical
decisions in bioethical contexts. The document makes four particularly relevant points:

- Respect for human dignity means that the 'interests and welfare of the
  individual should have priority over the sole interest of science or society'
  (Article 3).
- Human beings are fundamentally equal in dignity (moral worth), and for
  this reason should be treated 'justly and equitably' (Article 10).
- Any kind of discrimination against an individual or group constitutes a
  violation of human dignity (Article 11).
- At the same time, no cultural practices or beliefs may be appealed to justify
  violations of the dignity of the human individual.

Each of these points, in different ways, emphasises the worth of the individual
over any value that may be attributed to the group. They also emphasise the
fundamental equality of the worth between individuals.

Abortion, end-of-life decisions and appeals to human dignity

The tension between competing rights claims (between the individual and a group, as well as between individuals) is a feature of two controversies that have been significant in the development of the concept of human dignity in health-care ethics: abortion and end-of-life decisions. Because the concept of human dignity has become embedded in contemporary rights language as the basis of human rights, ethical language – especially where there are legal implications – also often uses the concepts of rights and dignity. However, since international human rights law presents dignity as the basis of human rights (UN, 1966a: Preamble), it means that competing rights claims often end up appealing to what appears to be the same basic principle.

In the case of abortion, the latter half of the twentieth century was characterised by debates between so-called pro-choice and pro-life positions. An extreme version of the pro-choice argument might be that a woman has the right to autonomous control over her body, and especially its reproductive capacities. An extreme version of the pro-life argument might be that every human being has a right to life, and therefore abortion (which constitutes directly ending a human life) at any stage of the pregnancy is always morally wrong. When asked to provide a justification for a woman's right to choose or the developing foetus's right to life, both sides may appeal to the concept of dignity, as enshrined in rights documents, to make their argument: to deny a woman the right to make autonomous choices about her body would violate her dignity; to end the life of the unborn child would violate its dignity. This is further complicated by seeming contradictions in human rights law. The UDHR states in Article 1 that all human beings are *born* with dignity. This could strengthen the so-called pro-choice case because it might be argued that the unborn foetus has no dignity. Yet international law has also set some precedents for human rights and protection of the unborn. This can be seen in the provision dealing with capital punishment in the International Covenant on Civil and Political Rights (UN, 1966a), which states, 'Sentence of death shall not be imposed for crimes committed by persons below eighteen years of age and shall not be carried out on pregnant women' (Article 6.5). Since a state may only execute a woman when she is not pregnant, there would seem to be an explicit recognition in international law that human rights – or at the very least, the right to life – should also be extended to humans who already exist but have not yet been born. Note that the appeals to dignity in the abortion debates have also paved the way for similar appeals with respect to other biomedical ethical issues surrounding early-stage human life – such as in-vitro fertilisation (IVF), pre-natal genetic testing, cloning, embryonic stem-cell research and so on.

In the case of end-of-life decisions, one might say that there are also two poles (though the full range of views is more complex). It could be argued that everyone has a right to 'die with dignity'. The final stages of life can be humiliating, as well as painful. People may lose control of their mental and physical capacities, and feel like a burden on others. It could be argued that this is a state of indignity, unworthy of a human person. To deny people the right to choose when and how to end their lives could be seen as constituting a violation of dignity because it condemns them to an undignified life, as well as denying their autonomy. Conversely, it could be argued that all human life has an inherent dignity or worth, and that to end any human life – including one's own – constitutes a violation of that inherent worth, and hence a violation of human dignity. Appeals to dignity with regard to end-of-life decisions are related to similar appeals in other areas. These include any cases where the degrees of self-control and autonomy are at stake, such as the treatment of temporarily incapacitated patients, aged care, the rights of people living with severe disabilities and the termination of pregnancies where there would be a high risk of disability for the child.

Controversies regarding the meaning and relevance of human dignity

The abortion and end-of-life debates illustrate the problem of 'dignity talk'. Dignity talk involves two or more interlocutors making competing rights claims to justify different courses of action by appealing to the same founda- tional principle – respect for human dignity – as a sort of argument-winning trump card. If human dignity is the basis of a particular right, then to deny that right appears to violate human dignity. The result is a stalemate, with neither side willing to give up its apparent moral high ground: that they are best respecting human dignity.

One reason for this may be that the use of the concept of dignity in human rights discourse might itself be ambiguous. Consider the following: human dignity, dignity of the human person, dignity of the person. Though, in each of these expressions, *dignity* might appear to refer to the same thing, it could be argued that there is a difference in meaning that hinges on what one understands by the concept of person.

In moral philosophy, and in law, persons are distinguished from property or objects. Persons have rights and duties; property cannot bear rights or exercise duties. It is for this reason that the law recognises the unjustified, intentional killing of a person as murder, but does not recognise the killing of cattle as murder.

Human dignity versus the dignity of the human person

Is it possible to be a member of the human species and not be a person? Regrettably, this question has been answered in the affirmative in the past, and some human beings are denied the rights of personhood in many contexts today. Slaves, though members of the human species, were not regarded as persons under the law, but rather as property. Women have been denied the full status of persons, and consequently the right to political participation. It was not until 1971 that women were given the right to vote in Switzerland. Children are still denied full legal personhood until they reach the age of majority. And some people still think it is acceptable to use force on a child that might constitute assault on an adult. It should be clear now why it was necessary for the UN to explicitly declare the equal dignity and rights of all members of the human species who were previously denied the status of persons either in law or in practice.

This sort of discrimination against certain members of the human species has been possible because, since antiquity, personhood has been associated with the possession and/or expression of particular capacities. Human beings who were deemed not to possess, or not to possess fully, certain capacities were denied the status of persons. Chief among these capacities is the ability to reason, or rationality. For example, in his *Nicomachean Ethics*, Aristotle (384–322 BCE) describes 'man' as a rational animal, and the proper function of 'man' as activity in accordance with rationality (1098a, 3–7, 1102b). In his *Politics*, Aristotle (1943) argues that the full realisation of rationality is expressed in the citizen, i.e., the bearer of rights and obligations in the city-state. Labourers, foreigners, women, slaves and children were excluded from being citizens.

According to Aristotle, this is because, 'the slave has no deliberative faculty at all; the woman has, but it is without authority, and the child has, but it is immature' (1260a, 11–14).

The association of personhood with rationality continues through the history of Western philosophy and theology in the work of highly influential thinkers such as St Thomas Aquinas and Immanuel Kant, and on into the present day. Note that even Article 1 of the UDHR seems to associate reason and the capacity to make informed moral decisions (conscience) with the notion of dignity.

Consequently, if one emphasises as the basic ethical criterion the dignity of human persons (as the 1945 UN Charter does), rather than human dignity, then, depending on how one understands 'person', 'rationality' and the possession of this capacity, it becomes possible to make a distinction between the moral worth of human persons and other members of the human species. For example, one might argue that human embryos do not possess rationality (though they may have a potential to possess it), and are therefore not persons or fully persons. One might make similar arguments with regard to human beings with severe mental disabilities or those in a persistent vegetative state.

Simply associating dignity with species membership, however, also poses several ethical challenges. For example, what should be done with frozen human embryos left over from IVF processes? Genetically speaking, each of these constitutes a unique member of the human species and would, therefore, according to a pure species membership argument for dignity, be entitled to treatment as persons of equal dignity. A simple thought experiment quickly illustrates the challenges of trying to maintain this position. Who would you save if an IVF laboratory were on fire – the laboratory technician or the frozen embryos?

Another difficult case is that of an anencephalic infant. If the worth of the individual is consequent upon its being a member of the human species alone, then it is entitled to the rights of all other human individuals, including life, food, shelter and so on. This would mean that babies born with this condition would have to be kept alive using artificial life support. Even in Catholic biomedical ethics, where dignity and species membership are frequently strongly associated to oppose abortion, an appeal is made to futility and the notion of disproportionate means to argue against the provision life support in such cases (O'Rourke & DeBlois, 1994). Yet this implies that species member-ship alone is not an adequate criterion for human dignity, and that other factors – such as the child's potential to develop sufficient mental capacity to live some sort of 'personal' life – must be taken into account.

The link between rationality, personhood and dignity can also be seen in the principle of respect for autonomy (Beauchamp & Childress, 2013), which is the ability of patients to make free, rational choices concerning their own interests and desires. This principle is applied by obtaining informed consent. Recalling the power imbalances in healthcare contexts, how well this practice respects autonomy – and hence personal dignity – is debatable. It is difficult to determine whether the information provided is understood or adequate. Moreover, there may be an assumption that consent should be given because the healthcare practitioner supposedly has the patient's best interests at heart, or speaks from a position of authority. This can put patients under pressure to consent to whatever the healthcare practitioner advises, even if they do not feel adequately informed. In other words, although it might appear as if autonomy is being respected, in practice the principle of beneficence – that is, to act in the patient's best interests – may be the dominant principle. This paves the way for the argument that certain patients cannot or do not know what is in their best interests, that they are making irrational choices and that respect for autonomy should be overridden by the principle of beneficence.

The principle of beneficence, then, may have more to do with respecting *human dignity* than respecting the *dignity of human persons*. It may assume that not all human beings are fully persons – that is, always capable of making rational decisions – but that their humanity, which implies certain interests beyond those that they subjectively express, should be respected by acting in these supposed best interests. (This, of course, does not necessarily imply that respecting human dignity so understood means disrespecting the dignity of human persons). So, in the end-of-life debates, for example, one might say that there is a tension between the principle of autonomy (dignity of human persons) and the principle of beneficence (human dignity). The former seems to support the idea that a person should be allowed to choose how to end their *own* life; the latter (usually) resists it. The latter may, however, support the ending of life (or at least 'letting die') where it is deemed to be in the patient's best interests or in the absence of any potential for interests (cf. the anencephalic child above). The problem here is that an argument could be made that this should be done even if it is against the patient's will – hence the need to counter the principle of beneficence with respect for autonomy.

Dignity of the human person versus dignity of the person

The examples of frozen human embryos and anencephalic neonates presented above raise an additional issue with respect to dignity, capacities and species membership. If personhood, and hence dignity, is associated with certain capacities and not species membership, then not only is it conceivable that not all humans are persons, but also that not all persons are human (Singer, 2009).

If one includes infants and people with mental disabilities as persons with full dignity, then one could also include those animals with intellectual capacities at least on a par with infants or people with mental disabilities as persons worthy of at least the same amount of respect. Conversely, if animals possessing such capacities are considered unworthy of being treated as persons, then human beings with diminished capacities could also be treated like these animals – for example, for the purposes of medical experimentation. Assuming that the latter is at the very least an unpalatable option for most people, and certainly counter to the spirit of the rights declarations mentioned above, this raises serious ethical questions regarding the slaughter of billions of animals for food, as well as their use in experimentation and production of medicines. Anything else is open to the charge of speciesism (Singer, 2009) – that is, an unjustifiable discrimination against animals that, although they have capacities similar to certain human beings, do not belong to the human species.

If, however, one maintains that species membership is morally significant, then this raises ethical questions regarding the global distribution of healthcare resources. Billions of dollars are spent on the care of companion animals while millions of humans die from preventable diseases every year.

Human dignity versus my dignity

Affirming human dignity in a generic, third-person sense is valuable and necessary to ensure just and ethical treatment of patients and staff in healthcare settings. However, it is of little value if this is not realised as a healthy sense of one's own worth as a human individual (Nussbaum, 2008). Unsurprisingly, therefore, debates about dignity in healthcare often have more to do with a first-person sense of the word *dignity*. Here, dignity has to do with one's own sense of self-worth: the sense that one is being respected, and that one does not have a good reason to feel humiliated (Margalit, 1996).

A patient who is being treated like a number, or like an 'in-valid', has cause to claim that their dignity is not being respected. A healthcare practitioner, too, may feel that their dignity is not being respected. In a world dominated by rights talk, and the commercialisation of public goods, patients can develop a strong sense of entitlement, either as tax-paying citizens or as fee-paying clients. Either way, this can lead to scenarios where healthcare practitioners are treated more like servants or human 'resources' than as human beings.

Perhaps more importantly, a patient may feel that they are losing their dignity. Consider a patient who is incontinent, or aware of the onset of dementia. Since dignity is frequently associated with capacities of self-control and agency, the sense that one is losing control, and one's identity, can negatively impact one's own sense of self-worth or dignity. To say to such a patient that, no matter what happens, they will always have their inherent dignity as a human being rings hollow, because it does not adequately address the patient's own experience of a perceived loss of dignity. Indeed, one could be accused of disregarding the patient's dignity if one does not take their personal sense of self-worth into account.

Navigating the tension between competing first-person claims to have one's dignity respected (for example, a patient and a practitioner) can be very challenging. It may be difficult to distinguish between subjective perceptions of deserved respect (first-person dignity) and objective reasons for claiming that one is not being respected (third-person dignity).

Human dignity versus the dignified human

Finally, there are times when dignity or worth is ascribed not on the basis of who (person) or what (member of the species) a human being is or thinks they may be (self-worth), but on the basis of what a person *does*. The previous examples of the incontinent patient and the 'in-valid' patient both help to illustrate this idea of dignity.

The incontinent patient has lost control of basic bodily functions. They can feel not only a loss of first-person dignity as a sense of self-worth (guilt), but also a loss of dignity in the eyes of others (shame) because of their apparently infantile behaviour. Recalling the reference to Aristotle above, childlike behaviour might imply a diminished rational capacity, and hence a loss of status as a dignified person in full control of one's rational capacities.

The disrespectful patient, too, could be said to be losing their dignity. This is not because their behaviour is infantile; rather, it is because it might be deemed unbecoming of a rational adult. If one holds that morally good behaviour results from rational deliberation, then one might also hold that morally bad behaviour demonstrates a lack of rational control, and a human individual not living up to their full dignity as a person. One might say that they are being unreasonable. Unlike the incontinent patient, who cannot control their behaviour, the implication here is that this patient could control their behaviour but they have chosen not to, and consequently have lost their dignity. Of course, there could be cases where people rationally choose to engage in immoral behaviour – or indeed do so on the basis of mistaken assumptions. The point being made here, however, is not about whether the person who is 'behaving badly' thinks they are behaving reasonably, but about how such 'bad behaviour' may be perceived by others.

Thus, in addition to the third-person idea of inherent dignity, and the first-person sense of my dignity, one could say that there is a second-person sense of dignity by which a person is deemed to have dignity (worth) to the degree that they behave in certain morally good, or at least socially acceptable, ways.

Rethinking human dignity: The multi-dimensionality of the human individual

The previous section demonstrated how different understandings of human dignity, and their relationship to the concept of personhood, can contribute to the problem of dignity talk: though the two sides of a debate seem both to be basing their claims on dignity, they are in fact basing their claims on different features of being human. Moreover, none of the possible bases for human dignity is patently false. It is true to say that human beings belong to a specific species, are (as a species) capable of rational thought, can develop a sense of pride or self-worth and live in societies that consider some forms of behaviour to be morally better than others. It is also true to say that each of these features is good – that is, has worth – and it is morally meaningful to speak of them as such.

The reduction of dignity to the affirmation of the worth of a single feature of being human loses sight of the reason why the concept of human dignity found its way into our ethical discourse in the first place – namely, as a response to atrocities that clearly denied the worth, importance and meaningfulness of human individuals – and the basic and useful assertion that there is some special worth that inheres in being human that makes an ethical claim on others not to treat one merely as an object, a dispensable thing. It is in a retrieval of this basic assertion that the solution to the problem of dignity talk lies.

Since the original intention of human dignity (as enshrined in rights documents) was to affirm the worth of human individuals, we must consider what we mean by human individuals. A human individual cannot be reduced to a single feature of being human. Therefore, it makes little sense to try to ground human worth in a single feature of being human. Rather, to speak meaningfully of human dignity is to speak of the worth of each individual as a multi-dimensional whole, and it is this whole that is, properly speaking, a person.

The component dimensions of human dignity model

The component dimensions of human dignity model (Table 4.1) offers a way to understand dignity as affirming the worth of the human person as a multi-dimensional whole (Kirchhoffer, 2009, 2013). Because it takes multiple bases of dignity into account, it also offers an interpretive framework through which differing claims in cases of dignity talk can more clearly be understood, and the normative justifiability of claims can be evaluated. Though this model may not always be able to tell us what the best ethical solution is in a particular case, it helps to identify those solutions that are unjustifiable, and promotes the continued search for better solutions that further the dignity of the human person as a whole.

The human person can be understood under four component dimensions. All of them must be taken into account to speak meaningfully of the notion of the dignity of a human individual.

TABLE 4.1 *The component dimensions of human dignity model*

COMPONENT DIMENSION	COMPLEMENTARY DUALITY	
	Already	Not yet
Existential	Have (potential)	Acquire (fulfilment)
Cognitive-affective	Inherent worth	Self-worth
Behavioural	Moral good	Morally good
Social	Others' dignity	My dignity

- The *existential component dimension* affirms that a human person is a particular existing embodied subject with the capacity to think, feel and act in a unique way in a unique set of relationships over time. It is the worth, the dignity of this particular bodily being in the world, that should be the focus of ethical reflection and action.

- The *cognitive-affective dimension* affirms that a human person is a subject who is capable of thinking (cognitive) and feeling (affective) in a particularly human way. In grammar, the subject is the noun that performs the action in a sentence – for example, 'I' is the subject of the sentence, 'I write.' This dimension affirms that a human person is an 'I', not merely the object of the actions performed by others. To affirm the idea that a human person is a subject is to affirm a particular set of capacities that make it possible to be a human being, rather than some other kind of being. Note that these capacities should not be limited to rationality. Emotion, or affect, is also integral to our self-awareness, and to our moral reflection and behaviour. We can feel that something is right or wrong; we can feel good or bad about ourselves. We can reason about a situation, make a free choice based on that reasoning and act on that choice, but we also have the capacity to love, even when this seems unreasonable (Farley, 1993). Martha Nussbaum (2000) proposes a set that includes life, bodily health, bodily integrity, senses, imagination and thought, emotions, practical reason, affiliation, other species, play, and material and political control over one's environment. These capacities may not always be expressed, and their development is heavily dependent on environmental factors and the opportunities that exist to develop them. If a person lives in a place where staying alive is difficult, the opportunities for development of other capacities may be limited. Nonetheless, their actual expression is not necessary to affirm their existence as a basic feature of human existence. That they exist in particular individuals constitutes a potential for their realisation in that individual.

- The *behavioural component dimension* affirms that the human person is an acting subject. Not only do we think and feel – which are internal actions – we also act outwardly in the world. Some of our actions are unconscious. We do not usually need to choose to breathe, for example. However, those actions that are consciously chosen or willed have the potential to be moral actions – that is, behaviours about which we can make judgements regarding their moral rightness or wrongness.

- The *social component dimension* affirms that human beings are always already in relationship with other human beings and with the world. We do not exist, think, feel or act apart from this fundamental relatedness. Moreover, our relationships are unique: no persons share the exact same relationships. Our moral behaviour as thinking, feeling and acting subjects is initiated by, and takes place in and through, our experiences of these relationships.

Since dignity refers to the worth of this human whole, dignity can likewise be understood in a multi-dimensional way. That is, instead of separating alternative bases for dignity as in the previous section (dignity is *either* in this feature *or* that feature of the human individual), it is possible to talk about the worth of different aspects of the human person that all need to be taken into account if one is to take seriously the worth of the whole (*both* this feature *and* that feature are integral to dignity). This makes sense given the previous observation that none of the bases offered for dignity is patently false, and they are all good things in themselves. In other words, human individuals do not possess dignity because they are members of the human species, or because they possess certain capacities, or because they have a sense of self-worth, or because they behave in a certain way. Instead, human individuals have dignity because they are members of a particular species that is characterised by a particular set of capacities, which are realised in living a meaningful life through their moral engagement with others and the world around them. When talking about dignity, each of the component dimensions is constituted by a complementary duality. These are two aspects of dignity that say slightly different things about dignity, which is why they are termed a duality. Nevertheless, both are necessary for a proper understanding of dignity with respect to a particular component dimension, and are therefore complementary (both ... and). For every component dimension, there is a pole of the duality that is already, and a pole of the duality that is not yet. The already pole contains features of dignity that are always already present and are unchanging. The not yet pole contains those aspects of dignity that can change, where dignity is something that can be acquired or realised, as well as something that can be violated or lost.

Every human person (properly understood in the multi-dimensional sense laid out here) exists as a particular being. From the moment when this person comes into being as a person to the moment they die, they exist as the same unchanging being. So someone might say they are the same person they have always been. But at the same time, because they are a person in relationship to the world, others and time, they change over time. So they might also say that they are not the same person they were at the age of 10. At the existential level, therefore, dignity is something that human persons both always already *have* because they exist, and something that they can *acquire* or lose because they exist as embodied subjects situated in time-bound or historical relationships.

At the cognitive-affective level, a particularly human set of capacities provides human persons with the potential to live meaningful lives as embodied subjects. By virtue of this potential to live a meaningful life, all human persons already have *inherent worth* (third-person dignity), regardless of whether this potential has yet been fulfilled in any way. At the same time, we have seen that it can ring hollow to affirm one's dignity if one does not have a conscious appreciation of one's own worth (first-person dignity). The person will therefore use their capacities to acquire a conscious sense of *self-worth* by living a meaningful life.

At the behavioural level, dignity – both as inherent worth and as self-worth – is a *moral good*. This means that dignity is an end or good in itself. It is something that should be the goal of morally good behaviour, and never merely a means (Kant, 2002). At the same time, we speak of the dignity of the *morally good*. These are people we think have behaved in a 'dignified' manner – that is, they have behaved in a morally good way that realises their inherent potential to live a meaningful life. Since having one's worth affirmed by others (second-person dignity) can help to affirm one's own sense of self-worth (first-person dignity), dignity as self-worth is partly acquired through engaging in behaviour that one subjectively believes to be morally good. Since dignity, both as inherent worth and as self-worth, is itself a moral good, engaging in behaviour that one subjectively believes furthers one's own sense of self-worth, as well as behaviour that one believes protects the inherent worth or self-worth of others, could be subjectively interpreted as morally good behaviour, and hence enhance one's sense of one's own dignity, even if this is not objectively morally good.

The social component dimension helps us to see whether what one subjectively believes to be morally good behaviour in an effort to realise one's own dignity as a sense of self-worth, as well as one's understanding of self-worth, really are objectively morally good, or at least not morally bad. As I seek to realise *my dignity* as a sense of self-worth, I must take into account that since dignity is a moral good, neither my understanding of self-worth, nor the behaviours in which I engage to achieve it, are morally justifiable if they depend on violating the moral good of *others' dignity*. Any behaviour or understanding of self-worth that appears to increase one's own self-worth to the detriment of the moral good of others' inherent worth is morally wrong because, by undermining others' inherent worth, I am also denying my own inherent worth. I cannot expect to be treated with dignity if I deny the basic premise on which this claim exists. This is the most rationally defensible way to understand the principle of respect for autonomy. There may, however, be occasions where limiting others' dignity as self-worth is morally licit where the others' sense of self-worth is itself dependent on the violation of others' inherent dignity. An unjustifiable sense of entitlement on the part of an aggressive patient does not require respect, but one still has to respect the worth of that patient that inheres in his potential to actually be a good person living a meaningful and dignified life, despite the present circumstances. This offers a way to understand the principle of beneficence and its relation to that of autonomy. Since the dignity of all human persons has clearly not been realised, my dignity also remains *not yet* realised.

This multi-dimensional understanding of human dignity resists the reduction of the human person to one particular feature. Thus any claim that dignity rests solely in species membership or in rationality is refuted, as is any claim that it rests solely on a person's own subjective desires or on some imposition of what society thinks a person should desire. However, each of these values still must be treated in relation to the dignity of the human whole. Understood in this multi-dimensional way, dignity is an end towards which we can strive in our ethical and political deliberation and behaviour. Instead of being a debate-ending trump card, human dignity invites us to look carefully at what it means to be human, and to see that the realisation of our own dignity, and the living of a meaningful life, require us to take the dignity of others as multi-dimensional meaning-seeking and meaning-making wholes seriously.

Reflective exercises

4.1 In this chapter, various international human rights documents have been presented. Map out a historical timeline for each of these documents. What are some of the international cultural or socio-political factors that may have influenced the development of each of these documents?

4.2 In 2005, the United Nations presented its Universal Declaration on Bioethics. Undertake a literature search and review this document.

- What are some of the key aims of this document, and how do these aims relate to the affirmation of human dignity in the provision of healthcare?
- What are some of the national healthcare legislative frameworks, health professional codes or position statements that would support the four relevant points in the declaration raised in this chapter?

4.3 This chapter has argued that there are some problems with what is termed 'dignity talk'. In this discussion, it is suggested that, due to ambiguous language in human rights discourse, there are conflicting arguments that form part of this 'talk'. Summarise each of these 'versus' arguments, and provide an example from your own clinical practice where this ambiguous discourse on human dignity may adversely impact upon the patient in your care or that of the health professional.

4.4 This chapter has presented a new way to view human dignity through acknowledging the multi-dimensionality of the human person. In Table 4.1, the author offers four component dimensions of human dignity.

- What are the key dimensions to each of the four components as a way to understanding dignity?
- What role does 'time' play in the model?
- Using the model, and especially its emphasis on taking the human person as a multi-dimensional whole into account, reconsider the examples raised in each of the 'versus' arguments. How might this multi-dimensional understanding of the human person and their dignity help to analyse these ethical issues? Remember to look for 'both ... and' type solutions rather than 'either ... or' distinctions. The example of the aggressive patient in the penultimate paragraph illustrates how you might do this.
- What are the benefits or limitations of adopting such a model in clinical practice, from a patient, healthcare provider or institutional perspective?

Notes

1. I use 'individuals' rather than 'persons' or 'beings' so as to avoid the problems that have arisen in the case of the two latter terms. These will be discussed below. I also use individual to underscore the point that it is each human who counts as having dignity, not simply humanity as a collective

concept. The latter would pave the way to utilitarian rationalisation that would enable us to deny the dignity of individuals for the good of the whole.

2. Compare this with the definition offered by Cicero in *De Inventione* 2.166 mentioned above.

References

Aristotle (1943). *Aristotle's Politics*, trans. B. Jowett. New York: Modern Library.

—— (1976 [1098]). *Nichomachean Ethics*, trans. J. A. K. Thompson. Harmondsworth: Penguin.

Beauchamp, T. L. & Childress, J. F. (2013). *Principles of biomedical ethics* (7th ed.). New York: Oxford University Press.

Cicero (1989). *De Inventione*. New York: Loeb.

Farley, M. A. (1993). A feminist version of respect for persons. *Journal of Feminist Studies in Religion*, 9(1–2): 183–98.

Kant, I. (2002 [1785]). *Groundwork for the metaphysics of morals*, trans. and ed. A. W. Wood. New Haven, CT: Yale University Press.

Kirchhoffer, D. G. (2009). Become what you are: On the value of the concept of human dignity as an ethical criterion in light of contemporary critiques. *Bijdragen*, 70(1): 45–66.

—— (2013). *Human dignity in contemporary ethics*. Amherst, NY: Teneo Press.

Margalit, A. (1996). *The decent society*, trans. N. Goldblum. Cambridge, MA: Harvard University Press.

Nussbaum, M. (2000). *Women and human development: The capabilities approach*. Cambridge: Cambridge University Press.

—— (2008). Human dignity and political entitlements. In President's Council of Bioethics (ed.), *Human dignity and bioethics: Essays commissioned by the President's Council on Bioethics*. Washington, DC: President's Council of Bioethics.

O'Rourke, K. & DeBlois, J. (1994). Induced delivery of anencephalic fetuses: A response to James L. Walsh and Moira M. McQueen. *Kennedy Institute of Ethics Journal*, 4(1): 47–53.

Singer, P. (2009). Speciesism and moral status. *Metaphilosophy*, 40(3/4): 567–81.

United Nations (UN) (1945) Charter of the United Nations Organisation.

—— (1948) Universal Declaration of Human Rights.

—— (1965) International Convention on the Elimination of All Forms of Racial Discrimination.

—— (1966a) International Covenant on Civil and Political Rights.

—— (1966b) International Covenant on Economic, Social and Cultural Rights.

—— (1979) Convention on the Elimination of All Forms of Discrimination Against Women.

—— (1984) Convention against Torture and Other Cruel, Inhuman or

Degrading Treatment or Punishment.

—— (1989) Convention on the Rights of the Child.

—— (1990) International Convention on the Protection of the Rights of All Migrant Workers and Members of Their Families.

—— (2005) Universal Declaration on Bioethics and Human Rights.

—— (2006) Convention on the Rights of Persons with Disabilities.

5 Empathy and care

Jānis (John) Ozoliņš

Empathy for the patient is a key attribute that is much prized in the healthcare professional. It is much harder, however, to specify what empathy is. It is to be distinguished from sympathy and compassion, as well as sentimentality. This chapter will explore the nature of empathy, drawing on the work of Edith Stein (1989). Care is central to healthcare but, in view of the discussion on empathy presented, this chapter will take a look at the ethics of care. The ethics of care argues for the importance of contextualising the relationships between care-givers and care-receivers.

The great advances in medical technology and the discovery of new, powerful drugs in recent times have led to a belief that almost all diseases and health problems can be treated efficaciously. We are told that the frontiers of what is medically possible are continually being pushed back, and that medical advances in areas such as nanotechnology and stem cell research promise to be able to treat currently incurable diseases. These advances are truly exciting, but healthcare is much more than the treatment of bodies that have succumbed to disease, or suffer from some disability. It is a truism to say that healthcare professionals do not treat bodies, but persons. Human beings who are suffering from health problems need much more than simply attention paid to their physical needs; they also need comfort and reassurance. Furthermore, it is also recognised that they need to have their psychological and spiritual needs met. In the healthcare setting, these needs are recognised through the provision of counselling and chaplaincy services. This, however, does not mean that the individual healthcare professional – such as a doctor or nurse – is relieved of a responsibility to treat patients as people by an assumption that the comforting and reassurance are the jobs of other members of the healthcare team.

Physicians and healthcare workers themselves recognise that medical technology has improved their ability to detect cancers, tumours and abnormalities that cause disease and suffering for patients. 'Imaging' – that is, x-rays, CT scans, ultrasounds and MRIs – has enabled early detection of various problems – such as, for example, tumours of the pancreas that can be removed before they become cancerous. In the past, physicians only had 'barium meals' to provide evidence of cancers, often too late to make a difference to the survival of the patient. Now CT scans and MRIs can provide early warning of problems. Paradoxically, however, it also means that various abnormalities that have little or no significance are also detected, and this requires physicians not only to see what the image depicts, but to also listen carefully to their patients when they talk about their symptoms. This is important for two reasons: first, to ensure that the detected abnormalities actually *are* the cause of the patients' health problems; and second, to provide reassurance and comfort to them in their suffering. It is easy to see the image on the screen, but far harder to listen to patients, make a correct diagnosis and empathise with them in their anguish at the explanation of their condition (Spiro, 2007).

Empathy, care and ethics

Before we consider what might be meant by empathy, a prior question is whether it is necessary for healthcare workers to empathise with their patients. There are many demands on healthcare workers to be efficient in their use of medical resources, to make correct judgements about diagnoses and treatments, and to maintain their professional knowledge of new techniques and technologies. Shiftwork and long hours in healthcare systems, as well as the demand to contain the costs of healthcare by minimising hospital stays and treatment times, leaves little time for healthcare professionals to be empathetic. Moreover, describing patients as clients, customers or consumers of healthcare, and healthcare professionals as healthcare providers, reduces the interaction between patients and healthcare professionals to one in which the basic requirement is the provision of the agreed service. Just as a shopkeeper is not obliged to do more than provide the goods that we have selected and to give us the correct change, so too a healthcare professional, under what we shall label as the customer view, does not need to do more than provide the service that has been demanded. Under this view, a healthcare provider acts ethically if they provide the described service to an acceptable standard. This fails to take into account the expectation that, in the healthcare context, the patient will be seen as a person with multi-dimensional needs.

Human beings are social creatures, and experience tells us that merely performing a medical procedure successfully is not enough – although, of course, we would be grateful to the socially inadequate but brilliant surgeon who saved our lives. Nonetheless, we would have reason to be offended if it was a matter of indifference to the surgeon whether we lived or died, and that all that mattered was the challenge of a difficult operation. It matters to us in a very personal way that our surgeon cares about our survival. Similarly, although it matters that our nurses are able to take our temperature, check our blood pressure and adjust our medications accurately, it also matters that they care about our well-being, and don't just see us as a customer to be served. It is this concern for the other that is at the heart of morality, and so empathy for the suffering other is central to our humanity. Empathy for the other is not an optional extra, but a moral response demanded of us in our dealings with our fellow human beings.

Care for others is central to the medical and healthcare professions, and care ethics is considered by many of its advocates to be a distinct ethical theory in its own right. The central concern for an ethics of care is the importance of attending to and meeting the needs of those others for whom we have responsibility. The parent of a child, for instance, has a moral responsibility to care for that child. In the case of children, their dependence on the care of others extends for many years. Similarly, when human beings are suffering from some malady, such as dementia, for which they require care, it is not just a matter of short-term intervention, but of long-term care and attention. In healthcare, there is an obvious responsibility to provide care to all those who require treatments for various health problems.

The ethics of care differs from other ethical theories in that, rather than focusing on the autonomous, independent and rational individual as central to moral theory, it focuses on the reality that human beings are dependent on each other for their well-being (Held, 2006). The ethics of care recognises our interdependence, and also that our prospects of human flourishing depend on others providing us with what we need to sustain our lives. Children need the care of parents, and human frailty in general means that many people will be dependent on the care of others at some time in their lives. Caring for others in need is a moral imperative since, given our interdependence, our own flourishing is inextricably tied to the flourishing of others, and human flourishing is good.

A second important dimension of an ethics of care is that, in focusing on human interdependence and relationality, it affirms the significance of the emotional dimension in our moral lives. Caring for others in their time of need is a matter of not merely attending to their physical needs, but also responding to them with sensitivity and empathy. This recognises that human beings need understanding, social support, love and affection, especially when they are afflicted by health and medical problems. Of course, not every emotion is appropriate: angrily and grumpily helping someone in need would be wrong, for example. In some instances, anger might be the right emotion to express – for example, when someone has not received the treatment they need and it is reasonable to express moral indignation. Sometimes expressions of emotions are inappropriate, but it is also the case that sometimes people do not know how to express the appropriate emotion. Grief is a good example of this. When someone has lost a loved one, many people have difficulty in responding to their loss. In the healthcare setting, very often the healthcare professional has to convey bad news, and being able to do this with compassion and empathy is essential in caring for the patient and for their family and loved ones. This highlights the importance of an education of the emotions.

Having the capacity to respond appropriately and sensitively by having the right emotional response is one element in an ethics of care. It is, however, not enough to make an appropriate response without any deep, whole-hearted empathetic identifying with the plight of the other and being there for them. That is, we should not be like an actor portraying a character who expresses an emotion, because this is playing a role and not real emotion. Acting does not involve genuine concern for the other; there needs to be appropriate intent or motivation to act for the right reasons. The ethics of care envisages the health-care practitioner responding authentically and suitably to the needs of the other in treating a particular health problem. It means being aware that patients have emotional, psychological and spiritual needs, which need to be handled with empathy and understanding. In providing healthcare, authentic concern for the other requires treating them as a human being like ourselves, and recognising their human dignity.

What is empathy?

Although it might seem that we have a good idea of what we mean by empathy, it is far from easy to characterise. For example, one perspective proposes that it is a feeling – almost 'magical' in medical practice – that brings passion and draws 'I and you' into 'I am you'. It grows from living and experience, and is looking out on the world from the point of view of the patient, trying to understand them better (Spiro, 2007: vii). Another perspective notes that it has many different definitions, but suggests that it is connected to sympathy, altruism, beneficence and compassion. It is suggested that it has come to imply tolerance, sensitivity and an ability to provide solace, care and comfort. Within the psychoanalytic literature, it has come to mean the projection of one person's consciousness onto another, and being affectively attuned to another person. It is regarded as a fundamental mode of human relatedness and, in agreement with the previous perspective, the recognition of the self in the other (Nadelson, 1993). Although this provides some explanation, we are still left with questions about what is meant by saying it is the recognition of the self in the other, since this could quite conceivably vary a great deal. A parent can see herself in her child because they are intimately related, but a young nurse may have considerable difficulty in recognising herself in an elderly male patient who is being treated for a self-induced, alcohol-related health problem. What is meant here is that the young nurse is able to recognise that the same humanity that is in her is also in the elderly male patient. If caring involves being affectively attuned to another person, and empathy implies actively seeking to ease their suffering, then it depends heavily on establishing unique relationships with each individual who is to be empathetically cared for.

If empathy is connected to sympathy, compassion, beneficence and altruism we need to be able to show how it is connected, as well as how it differs. If an empathetic nurse or medical practitioner is not the same as a sympathetic or compassionate one, it is not clear in what way. We value sympathy and compassion in others, so even if we do want to be treated by empathetic healthcare practitioners, we also want them to be sympathetic and compassionate. We also want nurses and healthcare practitioners to provide care that is beneficial, so we want them to exercise beneficence; it is therefore evident that it is connected to empathy, but it is equally obvious that it is not synonymous with it. This is because empathy for the other is what leads to beneficence – that is, beneficial treatment – but it is not itself the beneficial treatment. The connection of empathy to altruism is also unclear because it seems to suggest that the empathetic healthcare practitioner is expected to sacrifice their own well-being for us in some way. Though we might expect our loved ones to be prepared to look after us unselfishly, this seems to be an unreasonable expectation of our healthcare practitioners. Empathy for the other does have an element of altruism, however, since it is our empathetic recognition of the other that motivates us to put aside our own wants and desires to help the other. While this might not be altruism in the full sense of self-sacrifice, it suggests that empathy for the other leads us to do more for the other than is strictly required of us. A nurse might take a patient's blood pressure, but she might also chat to the patient while she does so, giving the patient a little more of her time than she needs to. Empathy is connected to other valued responses, and we need to be able to show what these are.

The concept of empathy has its roots in the translation of the German concept of *Einfühlung*,[1] and the term 'empathy' did not exist in English before the twentieth century (Slote, 2007). It has proved, and is acknowledged, to be a difficult concept to grasp (Hojat, 2007). Though we have suggested that it involves sensitivity, compassion and sympathy, it is none of these, since empathy is a broader concept and includes a cognitive component. Recognition of the cognitive component enables us to distinguish empathy from sympathy, since we can regard sympathy as an expression of feelings for another, whereas empathy also involves understanding the nature of another's emotional state, such as sorrow or joy (Hojat, 2007). Sympathy can also be taken to be more than openness to the emotions of the other, and to include a cognitive element insofar as sensitivity to another's feelings requires at least recognition of what it is that the other is feeling. This, however, does not translate into an understanding of those feelings, or into action on the part of the sympathiser. Because it requires openness to the other, sympathy enables the communication of feelings, but this need not translate into action.

Not only is empathy – a term coined by the psychologist E.B. Titchener (1909) – a difficult concept to grasp but, although a variety of definitions of empathy have been produced, there has been little consensus as to its meaning. The diverse definitions have had mixed success. Some have identified it with fellow-feeling, others with sympathy and losing oneself in the other. None of these has proved to be satisfactory. Among the earliest attempts to provide a clear description is that provided by Edith Stein (1989), a phenomenologist who wrote one of the first accounts of the concept. The phenomenological approach to providing an account of empathy is important, since it attempts to focus on what is common in our experience of empathy, bracketing out particular individual experiences. Stein's phenomenological treatment of empathy provides a means of distinguishing between sympathy, compassion and fellow-feeling, while acknowledging their role in our responses to each other. The phenomenologist focuses on the common elements of the experience of empathy that all individuals share, and so provides us with a clearer conception of it. This is vital if we accept that an empathetic concern for the other is crucial in healthcare.

Edith Stein

Edith Stein has been well known in Europe as a disciple of Husserl's, but it is only recently that her work has been available in English translation. Since her canonisation by the Catholic Church under her professed Carmelite name of

Theresa Benedicta of the Cross,[2] interest in her published work has grown. Her doctoral thesis, *On the Problem of Empathy*, is the only one of her works that was completed in an academic setting (Borden, 2003). Her analysis of empathy, drawing on the phenomenology of her teacher Edmund Husserl and also psychology, provides a systematic account of the concept. Her experience as a nurse during World War I suggests that it was no coincidence that she chose to study empathy.

Born into a Jewish family in 1891, Stein was one of the first women to be enrolled in a German university, commencing her studies in German studies, history and psychology at the Friedrich Wilhelm University in Breslau in 1910. In 1913, she moved to Göttingen to study under Husserl, completing her doctorate in 1916. In 1914, at the outbreak of World War I, she interrupted her studies, returned to Breslau and began medical training at All Saints Hospital. She then signed up for unconditional service with the Red Cross. Returning to Göttingen, while waiting for posting, she commenced her doctoral studies. Early in 1915, she received a call from the Red Cross and served for six months in a hospital for infectious diseases, receiving a medal of valour for her courage and service to the hospital. After completing her service to the Red Cross, she briefly returned to Breslau before following Husserl to Freiburg, where he had taken up a professorship. For a period after the completion of her doctorate, she worked with Husserl as his assistant, editing and preparing some of his work for publication. In choosing to write her dissertation on empathy, Stein was particularly interested in how we can have access to another's experience (Borden, 2003). That is, if we are to empathise with someone, we have to be able to determine what it is that they are experiencing before we are able to respond in an appropriate manner to their experience.

Although Stein had been born into a devout Jewish family, she lost interest in religion and became an atheist. While at Göttingen, she became interested in religion again, and a chance discovery of St Teresa of Avila's autobiography led her to convert to Catholicism and later to become a Carmelite nun. Although she was never to hold a formal academic post, she continued to write, producing a number of works in phenomenology, as well as a German translation of Thomas Aquinas's *De Veritate*. Although Stein had entered the Carmelites, this did not prevent the Nazis from rounding up her and her sister, Rosa (who had also entered the Carmelites), because they were Jews, and sending them to Auschwitz where they were gassed in 1942.

Stein's conception of empathy

MacIntyre (2006) comments that Stein begins her analysis of empathy by trying to identify what is primordial or primary in the experience of empathy – that is, what belongs to it as immediately given or transparently obvious, in contrast to what is mediated by kinds of experiences and so filtered through them. The difference here is between seeing something through a coloured lens and seeing it in plain light. For Stein, empathy is to be isolated from perceptions of various kinds: there is, in her view, something very basic about experiences of empathy. Stein (1989) says that if we exclude the physical world and the subject experiencing the world from our investigations, we are left with phenomena, and it is on these that she focuses. By this she means that we don't think about physical objects and we don't think about the identity of the person doing the experiencing, but just the unvarnished experiences or phenomena themselves. Merleau-Ponty (2007) – like Stein, a student of Husserl's – says that phenomenology tries to return to what is basic about what we experience, before we start to interpret and theorise about those experiences. In adopting the phenomenological approach, Stein seeks to identify what is basic about empathy, separated from all the other kinds of experiences that human beings have.

For the clinical psychologist, as well as the philosopher, phenomenology is attractive because it is an approach to understanding human beings that focuses on their unvarnished experiences – that is, the phenomena that form the content of those experiences. For example, in feelings of anger, the phenomenologists focus on what makes anger the experience that it is and is not – say, irritation. Concentration on the phenomena enables us to investigate questions such as what it is like to be a schizophrenic, to be compulsive, to feel suicidal, depressed, grief-stricken or joyful without complicating the picture with the particular individual who is having these experiences (Margulies, 1984). In short, phenomenology investigates the inner life of human beings by identifying the phenomena that are the primary components making their experiences. Experiences themselves are constructed out of phenomena and other experiences, biases, memories and ideas that serve to interpret the phenomena for the subject. In a sense, phenomena are our basic perceptions of the world before they become subjective. In the healthcare context, a phenomenological approach helps practitioners to be aware of being able to see that their experience of situations is overlaid with their own subjectivity. This awareness helps them to allow for their subjective experiences, biases and preconceptions, and to see the phenomena more objectively. A difficult patient's behaviour, for example, may not be simply because they are a difficult, cantankerous person, but be due to stress and fear that, if recognised, can be addressed. Phenomenology tries to provide a direct description of our experience as it is, without taking account of its psychological genesis, and the causal explanations that the scientist, the sociologist or the historian may be able to provide (Merleau-Ponty, 2007).

The notion of phenomenological reduction or bracketing that originated with and was refined by Husserl (2000) was the outcome of his rejection of all forms of psychologism – broadly speaking, the view that psychological techniques can be used to solve philosophical problems, particularly those to do with the human mind and consciousness. He also rejected naturalism – the view that problems of consciousness and of the mind can be solved using the methods of the natural sciences. Instead, Husserl says we should turn away from the natural world and focus instead on the life of our consciousness. That is, if we bracket out everything that is not the world as it is present to us in our consciousness, we are left with our own purely subjective understanding of the world – phenomena – but also with the realisation that we, as human beings, also experience ourselves as belonging to that world. The further task of the phenomenologist is to show that the different subjective experiences of the world nevertheless are eidetic experiences of the same world (Kockelmans, 1994). That is, although each individual experiences phenomena subjectively, they will have common features.

Phenomena form the basis of our relationship with the world. When we consider a phenomenon like a perception – one we are having in the here and now – our later memory of it will be different from what we experience now. Remembering that I felt joy is not the same as experiencing it now. An act of empathy is not a perception in the ordinary sense, and this is illustrated by considering an example. Stein (1989) asks us to consider what occurs when someone informs you that his brother has died and you become aware of his pain. Stein proposes that we should reflect on the nature of this awareness. It is not, she says, just a kind of outer perception, by which she means it is not a perception like seeing an object. We see trees, but we don't see pain. Nevertheless, we become aware of a person's sorrow, even though it is not conveyed by the words uttered. Neither, for that matter, is it something that is an inner perception – by which we mean a thought or idea which comes into our minds. It is primordial – that is, immediately given in experience in the same way that any other perception is; since our awareness of another's grief is an observation, the grief is not our grief. It is not, however, just an observation of external bodily movements, facial expressions that we label as grief. We are aware that it is the phenomenon of grief we observe. It is this awareness that what we observe is more than the observation of the outward manifestations that distinguishes empathy from perception.[3] Empathy is not like memory, expectation and fantasy, which are not primordial in the sense that ordinary perceptions are because they are recalled from within our minds. (Stein, 1989). These are all inner perceptions of our minds –we are aware of recalling our memories, fantasising about and imaging things. Recalling an experience of seeing the *Mona Lisa*, for example, is not the same as experiencing it here and now. Nor is fantasising that we are a famous rock star the same as actually being one. Empathy is more than just a recalling of our own feelings of grief and a kind of projection of this onto our observations of the grief of the other.

Nevertheless, MacIntyre (2006) says that our relationship to the feelings of others is analogous to our relationship to our own past feelings. I can put myself imaginatively in another's shoes and know they are experiencing joy, but this does not mean that I experience the joy that they are experiencing. He adds that Stein rejects Mill's explanation that we know our own feelings and thoughts directly, and those of others indirectly, through perceiving that they have the same bodily movements that we do when they express feelings and thoughts. Stein rejects this explanation because it supposes that we already know that others resemble us both in having an inner life like ours and expressing it in the same kind of way. Our relationship to the feelings of others is not indirect in the way Mill supposes. Stein (1989: 66) says that, 'An individual's movements are not given to us as merely mechanical movements'. This means that it is not just bodily movements with which we are presented, but an awareness of the emotions and feelings that the bodily movements express (MacIntyre, 2006).

When we are faced with someone's grief, we become aware of the grief itself, not just its expression. Both Husserl and Stein argue that we know directly when someone is in pain or is grief-stricken. The distinction that is being alluded to here is quite important, for empathetic awareness of someone's grief is not the same as perceiving that they are acting in a grief-stricken way. To be aware of the grief of another is to be aware of the phenomenon of grief as reaching much deeper into the soul of the other. Otherwise, a feigned grief of an actor playing a role would be expressing the same thing as real grief. Another way of seeing this is that we do not want our healthcarers to *pretend* to be empathetic; we want them to actually *be* empathetic. Genuine grief (or joy) is self-evidently something other than someone playing a role. Husserl remarks in the *Logical Investigations* that, 'Common sense credits us with perceptions even of other people's inner experiences: we "see" their anger, their pain, etc. Such talk is quite correct.' (Husserl, 2000: 277–8)

In empathising, our experience of empathetic grief or joy, for example, is an indirect experience, since it is not we who are actually experiencing the grief or joy itself. Leaving aside for the moment that it is we who are having an experience – a direct experience, which is of empathy – the content of what we experience is indirect. We become aware of the other person's grief or joy, and we empathise with them. The empathetic experience of grief or joy we experience is thus indirect, since our experience of it is dependent on our becoming aware of what the other is experiencing. It is the other's experience of grief or joy that prompts our own response – which is, in a manner of speaking, a reflection of the grief or joy of the other. It is in that sense that we can talk of empathy as a species of fellow-feeling. It is more than this, since there is also a cognitive understanding that what we are conscious of in the other is grief or joy, and not something else, and that our empathetic response is the appropriate one. Stein (1989) notes that we can live the other's joy, but we do not feel the primordial joy. The experience I have, however, is not the same as either remembering or imagining. It is something other than this and just as basic.

Stein (1989) explains that empathy is a kind of act of perceiving *sui generis*. It is the experience of a foreign consciousness, and it is in this third way (apart from memory and imagination) that human beings comprehend the psychic life of their fellows. It is through empathising with others that we comprehend the feelings of others, and we learn to distinguish between the different emotions that they are feeling. The difficulty, which Stein recognises, is that we still have some distance to go before we can be sure that we can identify the particular emotion someone is experiencing, and be able to respond empathetically in an appropriate manner to them.

This highlights the importance of the cognitive component of empathy, and why it differs from sympathy, which is an emotional response to another. First, unless we know what grief or joy is, we are unable to recognise what another is experiencing, much less respond to them empathetically in an appropriate way. Suppose a friend comes to us and joyfully tells us she has passed her exam. We can comprehend this joy empathetically, and become joyful over it ourselves, but we cannot do so unless we have an experience of joy in a similar kind of way. If we have had the joy of passing an exam, we can recall the memory of the joy and elation we felt, and so are able to enter empathetically into the joy of our friend. It is evident that we do not experience the joy directly, just as in the case of remembering, we do not directly experience the joy that we remember, but rather evoke feelings of joy through remembering the joy that we felt previously. Similarly, in empathetic joy, we do not feel the joy of the other person in the direct way that they do, but we feel real joy nevertheless through empathising with them (Stein, 1989: 14). Second, although we might be able to recognise what another is experiencing, an empathetic response also requires that we respond appropriately. It is not enough to recognise that someone is experiencing grief, and to feel sympathy; an empathetic response will be one in which we respond in an appropriate manner.

Stein (1989) contends that, through empathy, we come to experience the consciousness of others and respond to them appropriately. Though there are further questions to be asked about the ways in which we can experience foreign consciousnesses, it is evident that her conception of empathy leads us to look beyond mere bodily movement and mere emotion. The need to have a rich emotional life ourselves also leads us to look beyond the obvious and, in the healthcare context, to realise that patients have a rich, complex inner life that reflects their essential character. In empathising with them in their afflictions, we draw on our own experiences, and this implies being schooled to recognise and respond to others in an appropriate way. Seemingly odd behaviour, for example, may reflect deep-seated anxieties, longings and fears that cannot adequately be expressed by a brain and a body suffering from some malady, which are no longer responding in a way they should. In empathetic awareness, we are conscious that we need to look beyond the surface to discern what a suitable empathetic response should be.

Healthcare and empathy

Within the clinical setting, empathy is first a recognition that another is in pain or suffering, and second being able to respond in the appropriate manner. This demands a significant intellectual effort since, as we have already discussed, responding empathetically has a cognitive component. In being empathetic, the clinician does not experience the pain herself, since it is the patient's pain, but can empathise with the suffering that accompanies the pain. No clinician, after all, will – no matter how hard they try – be able to experience the pain and suffering of the patient in a direct way. Sympathy for the patient's pain and suffering involves feeling for the patient, but does not involve – as empathy does – appreciating the pain and suffering from within the perspective of the patient, without that pain and suffering being directly the clinician's own.

Although sympathy is a human response to human affliction, in the clinical setting it can cloud the healthcare practitioner's judgement, and so be a liability in treating a patient appropriately. In an empathetic response, however, the patient's state of pain and suffering is apprehended in an objectification of the experience in such a way that the clinician's response, while including an emotional component, is objective and appropriate.[4]

In our brief discussion of the ethics of care, we noted that human beings are social creatures, which means that they are dependent on one another for their well-being. Human beings cannot survive from childhood to adulthood without support from parents and other caregivers who guide them. Neither does dependence end on reaching adulthood. Human beings need each other, not only to provide the basic necessities of life, but also to provide companionship and affiliation. Being able to connect with one another is also a need of human beings.

The need for connectedness is another important element in healthcare. It has been widely recognised that making connections can be a major factor in the maintenance of health and well-being. Having the support of family and friends plays an important role in the prevention of disease and the mainte-nance of health (Hojat, 2007). Healthcare outcomes are enhanced if patients have good social support networks. Patients with heart disease have a better chance of survival if the healthcare practitioners and clinicians treating them recognise that it is not just the physical needs of patients that need to be attended to, but also their social, emotional and spiritual needs (Hojat, 2007). An empathetic response to patients by clinicians is a necessary component of good healthcare.

In treating patients, healthcare practitioners are called upon to respond in an empathetic way to them. This means that they are to treat the whole person, and patients are not to be divested of their humanity. Empathy is not an optional extra, but is a key element in healthcare practice. Within the ethics of care, human relationships are central, and so are our affective responses to each other. Empathy is crucial in the ethics of care because it ensures that the emotions that are part of our relationships with others are understood in the context of what constitutes a proper response to the other. Sympathy alone, for example, might enable us to feel the pain someone is experiencing, but not understand the suffering they are enduring. Empathy enables us to experience in an indirect way the phenomena that constitute their whole experience and to respond appropriately. It is vital that healthcare practitioners not only know the essential elements of their profession, but also know how to empathise with their patients.

Reflective exercises

5.1 In your own words, describe what you think are some of the character-istics of being empathic in the provision of healthcare. What are some of the barriers or limitations to providing such care in clinical practice?

5.2 What are the main differences between empathy, sympathy and compassion?

5.3 This chapter provides a definition of the 'ethics of care'. The reciprocal nature of care underpins this definition. Why is this so?

5.4 Generic terms such as clients, customers and health consumers have become part of the healthcare lexicon over the last decade, predominantly in response to the economic rationalisation of services. Reflect on the impact of such language on the understanding of empathy and care in your clinical area.

5.5 Healthcare practitioners should keep a 'professional distance' from their patients. Is such a position conducive for provision of empathic care?

5.6 Can we recognise an emotion that we have never felt? Suppose we have never experienced grief. Can we empathise with someone who is griev-ing? How would we know they are grieving? Discuss.

5.7 Review the discussion about Stein's analysis of empathy. Considering this understanding, can a healthcare professional truly empathise with a cognitively impaired patient, such as someone living with advanced dementia?

5.8 Only truly caring health professionals can care ethically for their patients. Discuss with relation to relationality and interdependence, two important dimensions in an ethic of care.

Notes

1. *Einfühlung*, roughly translated, means 'in feeling' or 'feeling into something'.

2. Edith Stein was canonised by Pope John Paul II on 11 October 1998. Gassed by the Nazis in Auschwitz in 1942, she has the distinction of being the first saint in 400 years to be canonised for being both a person of heroic virtue and a martyr.

3. Sharon Todd (2006) considers what the notion of 'feeling with' as opposed to 'being for' – Baumann's term for the commitment that one should have for the other – adds to the issue of determining moral values in her discussion of our relation to the other.

She notes that Stein's conception of empathy has a moral dimension, as we have already suggested. She locates the origins of the notion of 'fellow-feeling' in Adam Smith and David Hume; however, Stein's conception is more than fellow-feeling, since it has a profoundly moral dimension. Todd does not see empathy as providing a sufficient basis for ethical possibility, however (see Todd, 2006: 49–50, 62–3). Arguably, Todd has not considered Stein's analysis in sufficient detail. It is quite clear that Stein maintains a separation between the self and the other in her conception of empathy. Empathy is more than a 'being-for' since, although difference between the self and the other is maintained, empathetic understanding is a recognition of our ability to be in communion with one another.

4. Hojat (2007) provides a very useful table outlining the differences between sympathy and empathy. A key difference, he maintains, in agreement with Stein's analysis, is that empathy has a cognitive component. He says, for example, that in empathy, the healthcare practitioner understands the suffering of the patient, whereas in sympathy, she feels the patient's pain.

References

Borden, S. (2003). *Edith Stein*. London: Continuum.

Held, V. (2006). *The ethics of care: Personal, political and global.* Oxford: Oxford University Press.

Hojat, M. (2007). *Empathy in patient care: Antecedents, development, measurement and outcomes.* Dordrecht: Springer.

Husserl, E. (2000). *Logical investigations 1*, #7, trans J. N. Findlay. Amherst, NY: Humanity Books.

Kockelmans, J. (1994). *Edmund Husserl's phenomenology*. West Lafayette, IN: Purdue University Press.

MacIntyre, A. (2006). *Edith Stein: A philosophical prologue*. London: Continuum.

Margulies, A. (1984). Toward empathy: The uses of wonder. *American Journal of Psychiatry*, 141: 1025–33.

Merleau-Ponty, M. (2007). What is phenomenology? in T. Toadvine & L. Lawlor (eds), *The Merleau-Ponty Reader*. Evanston, IL: Northwestern University Press.

Nadelson, C. C. (1993). Ethics, empathy and gender in health care. *American Journal of Psychiatry*, 150: 1309–14.

Slote, M. (2007). *The ethics of care and empathy*. London: Routledge.

Spiro, H. (2007). Foreword. In M. Hojat, *Empathy in patient care: Antecedents, development, measurement and outcomes*. Dordrecht: Springer.

Stein, E. (1989). *On the problem of empathy* (3rd rev. ed.). Washington, DC: ICS Publications.

Titchener, E. B. (1909). *Lectures on the experimental psychology of the thought-processes*. New York: Macmillan.

Todd, S. (2006). *Learning from the other*. New York: SUNY Press.

6 Healthcare and virtue

Jānis (John) Ozoliņš

Virtue ethics is one of the major normative ethical theories, and has a very long history, having its origins, among other places, in the eudemonic ethics of Aristotle. Virtue ethics begins by considering the question of what is meant by the good for human beings and answers that it is to live a life of moral virtue. For Aristotle (1976), four cardinal moral virtues were required: courage, temperance, justice and prudence. Added to these in the Christian era are the theological virtues of faith, hope and charity, which also make a distinctive contribution to ethical decision-making in the healthcare context.

Character and virtue

The beginnings of virtue ethics can be found in reflecting on the kind of healthcare practitioner by whom we would like to be treated. If we are facing delicate brain surgery to alleviate a particular condition, we would want a good brain surgeon, not a poor one. Similarly, when we are later returned to the ward after a successful operation, we would want to be looked after by a competent nurse, rather than one who is incapable of performing their duties. This is true in every area of life. No one wants their MRI scans interpreted by an incompetent physician or to be represented by an inept lawyer. The slow lane at the checkout at the supermarket, where the checkout operator is bumbling and unskilled, is also to be avoided. In all these cases – as in every situation where we rely on the skills and competencies of others – we want those providing various services not simply to have some minimal competence, but to carry out their roles or activities well.

In these examples, our concern is that the brain surgeon, the nurse, the physician, lawyer and checkout operator are good at what they do. That is, they are competent and skilled at their jobs. Likewise, when we say of a football player that he is a good player, we mean at least that he is skilful, reads the play well and contributes to the success of his team on the field. In all these cases, good means the possession of certain abilities and capacities that enable individuals to carry out particular tasks and actions well. It is also apparent that we value the superior or competent performance of these tasks because it contributes in some way to our well-being. Surgery performed well leads to a return to health, competent nursing hastens our recovery and correct interpretation of MRI scans leads to the identification of possible internal problems that might threaten our health. An able lawyer and skilful checkout operator can save us time and relieve stress, making our lives easier. Being good at what they do enables them to contribute to our well-being.

Although being able to do something well is important, it is not the only good with which we are concerned. We are grateful if our surgeon has the skill in their hands to perform surgery well, but we are not likely to admire their possible poor bedside manner. Similarly, we are not likely to admire the nurse who is rude to and impatient with their patients, no matter how well they are able to insert a cannula into a vein. Professional codes of conduct provide guidelines about how healthcare practitioners should behave towards their patients in carrying out their duties, but they also include advice about how healthcare practitioners should act when they are not on duty. These codes of conduct are virtue orientated. For example, the Code of Professional Conduct for Nurses in Australia not only requires that nurses uphold exemplary standards of behaviour and reach required competency levels, but also that they should be exemplary in their private lives. Thus the code states that nurses ought not engage in such wrongful behaviour as sexual assault, theft and being drunk and disorderly in a public place (ANMC, 2008). The United Kingdom Nursing and Midwifery Council (2010) advises nursing and midwifery students that they must be of good character, and be honest and trustworthy. Being a good nurse or healthcare practitioner involves more than the skilful performance of the tasks required of the role; it includes being of good character, and this has something to do with our dispositions – that is, with how we are disposed to act.

We know what it means for someone to be a good healthcare practitioner in a certain field, since we can list the competencies required. We also know the reasons why practitioners need these competencies. The reason we should be of good character in our profession, however, is not so obvious. If an adulterous surgeon operates on us or a nurse with a weakness for alcohol and petty pilfering of hospital stationery nurses us, it is not clear that our treatment is affected by these character flaws. While it may not be so obvious how these character flaws affect our treatment, there are other character traits that, if our surgeon or nurse possessed them, might lead us to be more worried about our likely treatment. If those who were treating us were cruel, sadistic and heartless, for example, we would not be quite so sanguine about the irrelevance of character traits. This is because these character traits incline or dispose individuals to act according to these characteristics. A nurse who is cruel or sadistic will at best be unmoved by any pain and suffering she might inflict and, while she may perform her tasks competently, will not regard the alleviation of pain and suffering as integral to her role. It is reasonable to conclude that good character is a requirement for someone to be a good healthcare practitioner.

Informally, good character is demonstrated when individuals show themselves to be trustworthy, loyal and honest. The reason why having these kinds of dispositions demonstrates good character is related to the question of what it means to be a good human being. Just as we can recognise good surgery as surgery successfully performed, a good human being will be one who acts well, in accordance with what is required of a human being. What is required of a human being is that they fulfil their function as a human being – that is, they possess those traits and dispositions that enable them to reach their full potential. The proponent of virtue ethics proposes that a good human being is one who possesses the virtues, and it is possession of the virtues that leads us to say that someone is of good character. A good surgeon is therefore both competent in doing surgery and possesses the virtues.

Virtue ethics approaches moral philosophy differently from either the Kantians or utilitarians. It emphasises character and its development rather than the rules for performing one's duty or for the evaluation of the consequences of actions. Virtue ethicists are concerned, moreover, not with the question of what one ought to do in a given circumstance, but rather with the question of the sort of person that one *ought* to be. The primary and central moral judgements are about the character of persons who act. Virtuous persons are those who conduct themselves according to certain dispositions that enable them to pursue the good both for themselves and others. We need to consider how to determine what the virtues are, why they make us good persons, why the end of human beings is the good and how this relates to healthcare practice.

In recent decades, virtue ethics has emerged as a serious rival to deontological (Kantian) ethics and utilitarian ethics. One reason for this – particularly for healthcare practitioners – is that neither Kantian nor utilitarian ethics takes into account the particular sensitivities and responsibilities of professional roles. In both of these, a hallmark is impartiality in determining what moral action is to be chosen. Virtue ethics in contrast regards the character of the individual actor as central, and this will include human goods such as friendship (Oakley & Cocking, 2001). In the professional sphere, this means that not only is competence important, but so is the professional relationship between practitioners and patients. Characteristics such as kindness, patience and trustworthiness are crucial, and are vocational characteristics of healthcare service provision.

Approaches to virtue ethics

There are two main approaches taken by virtue ethicists to establish the account of the characters of good human beings: an Aristotelian approach where happiness is the end of human beings; and an approach in which it is the virtues themselves that are essential for human fulfilment, even though this does not necessarily lead to happiness. The first approach draws on Aristotle's view that the character of good human beings is determined by what we need, or what we are, as human beings. The virtues are the traits of character that human beings need in order to lead lives that are fully human – that is, flourishing lives in which there is fulfilment and contentment. The virtues are the traits of character that we need in order to live the flourishing, contented human lives that lead to happiness. Virtues such as kindness, trustworthiness and justice, because they interconnect with intrinsic goods such as courage, integrity, friendship and knowledge, are virtues because we cannot have a flourishing life without them. Together with the virtue of practical wisdom or prudence, the virtues are at least partly constitutive of happiness and hence, if happiness is the end of human life, intrinsically good elements of a good human life (Oakley & Cocking, 2001).

The second approach takes a different view of the virtues by arguing that what is central is the development of human capacities and character traits, irrespective of whether or not they lead to happiness. Happiness here seems to be taken to mean subjective pleasure or satisfaction. Love of knowledge, friendship and the satisfaction of achievement through work, for instance, count as virtues because they help us to realise our full potential as human beings, but they may not necessarily lead to much happiness for the individual (Oakley & Cocking, 2001). For example, a great artist may eke out a miserable existence, barely making a living, but nevertheless be fulfilled because, though their work is unrecognised as great art, they are aware that they have accomplished what they set out to do. They have developed their talents and abilities to the fullest capacity. Perhaps the artist's refusal to compromise their artistic standards may result in commissions for paintings being withdrawn, and so the artist's life is not a particularly easy one. In a real sense, such a person is prepared to suffer for their art. It is difficult to argue that the artist is happy in this suffering – that is, they do not take pleasure in it – but we can certainly see the virtue in someone's uncompromising integrity and devotion to their art.

The Aristotelian approach, however, has the advantage of providing a clearer justification for the pursuit of virtue, and understands happiness as being more than subjective pleasure or contentment. If the pursuit of virtue does not lead to happiness or contentment, however, then it is difficult to see why anyone would be motivated to be virtuous. Arguing that there is satisfaction to be gained from fulfilling our potential, despite it leaving us miserable, appears to appeal to some form of superior, rarefied contentment, which is arguably another mode of happiness. It is one thing to argue that the possession of virtue does not guarantee happiness, but quite another to argue that its possession is its own reward. The Aristotelian approach provides an answer to the question of what human beings are for, and happiness understood as human fulfilment through the possession of the virtues is lasting – unlike subjective pleasures. Human beings are created for lasting happiness and, as Thomas Aquinas, who develops and extends the Aristotelian account of the virtues, argues, human beings are made for God. That is, although the virtues will lead to (imperfect) happiness in this world, Aquinas (1981) says that the final end for human beings is to be with God.

Aristotle and the good for human beings

Aristotle regards ethics as being concerned with human action, and in particular with those actions that lead to the good. The good Aristotle regards as that which leads to a full, well-lived life, and the necessary ingredient in attaining such a life, is virtue. A central question is what Aristotle might mean by 'good', and this is the question he discusses at the beginning of Book I of the *Nichomachean Ethics* (1976).[1] He observes, however, that the various activities of human beings have a variety of ends, and so it is not at all clear from these what 'good' might encompass. For example, for a medical practitioner, the end is the health of their patients, for a military commander, it is victory and for an entrepreneur, it is wealth. All of these ends in some sense are all good, since it is what our activities are aiming towards. The question raised by Aristotle asks us about the sense in which we can say that all of these ends are good – that is, what do they share that makes them all good, yet completely different from each other? Aristotle responds by suggesting that our activities aim at some end that we ultimately want for its own sake, and for the sake of which we want all other ends. The final end for which we aim is the supreme good, and it is knowledge of what this consists that is of paramount importance to us for the conduct of our lives.

Aristotle sees what he is trying to do in the *Nichomachean Ethics* as closely tied to an understanding of politics, which for Aristotle is the science of understanding how human beings can live in community. Aristotle notes that while the welfare of the individual is of great importance, that of the community is of greater importance. He says that while it is good to secure individual good, what is far better is to secure what is good for the community (Aristotle, 1976). The good is not always what accords with the desires of the individual, and Aristotle clearly states that the good of the community may well override the good of the individual. Virtue cannot be practised in isolation. The central question for Aristotle is to give some account of what could be meant by the good, but it is the good in relation to a life lived well, and so for the individual it is a question of determining what is required in being able to live a successful life. It is also clear that many things we regard as good can lead to evil consequences – wealth can be squandered on indulging one's senses (gambling, sex, drugs) and we can be brought undone by our courage. Aristotle warns us about confusing being successful with having the wherewithal to be successful. Having wealth, courage, power or fame may be the ingredients for a successful life, but these things do not inevitably lead to a successful life, since it is how we use these in our daily activities that determines whether our lives will be successful or happy.

Aristotle notes that an essential ingredient in being able to lead a happy life is being able to make the right judgements about how to act, and the ability to do this will depend on having a good general education. In addition, this includes having the self-discipline to control one's feelings, for having knowledge is of no use if we are unable to control our impulses. Pursuing one's aims while under the influence of emotions, he says, will not be successful, since we will be blinded by them and unable to act rationally (Aristotle, 1976). While this does not tell us what it is to lead a happy life, it does suggest that certain kinds of lives can be ruled out from consideration. For example, a debauched life is ruled out by Aristotle's remarks about the need to control one's feelings; it is not, as far as he is concerned, a life worth living.

Lives worth living

The question of what kinds of lives are worth living is very important in the context of healthcare professions. Issues surrounding the treatment of terminally ill patients, for example, frequently centre on judgements about the kinds of lives that are worth living. The virtue ethicist will take a very different approach to answering this question from the utilitarian one. For the virtue ethicist, it is not a matter of a weighing of preferences, but a consideration of the good of the patient, irrespective of whether they have some rational reason for desiring death. While virtue ethicists might arrive at different responses about how end-of-life situations ought to be handled, all will agree that healthcare should aim at enabling human beings to lead flourishing lives. They will be guided by such virtues as compassion, honesty, conscientiousness, care, integrity and respectfulness. The question becomes not one about what kind of life is worth living, but about what is needed to bring about what is good for the patient (Oakley, 2013). In Aristotle's view, for those with sufficient independent means not to need to work, there are three main types of life worth living: a life of pleasure, a life of honour in political service and a contemplative life. The life of pleasure, he says, is inadequate, because it reduces persons to the level of animals – though many powerful and important people share a predilection for the pursuit of pleasure. Honour also depends on who confers the honour, and Aristotle suggests that the gaining of honour is generally pursued because it enables an individual to gain a good reputation, both in their own eyes and in the eyes of the community. Insofar as this is so, it appears that honour is pursued for a further good, not just for its own sake. This further good is not something like Plato's form of the good, but is success in life, and this is the only objective for human beings. This leaves the contemplative life.

The way is now open for us to pursue the analysis of what Aristotle means by success in life, which is what he considers to be happiness. As we have already noted in the examples above, for any particular human occupation, whether a person performs it well or not is determined by the proficiency with which that occupation is carried out. Hence, to use Aristotle's own example, a flautist will be considered a good flautist if they perform well – that is, if they carry out their function of playing the flute well. By analogy, the function of human beings is an activity of the soul that accords with a rational principle, which is to say that to live well a person has to be directed by a rational soul. Success in life – the best possible good for human beings – is therefore living one's life in a rational way, under the guidance of the best and most perfect kind of virtues of the rational soul. The judgement that a life has been successful can only be given on how an entire life has been lived – a person will be a happy person if they have lived their life virtuously, and enjoyed moderate good fortune all the days of their life. Until a life is over, Aristotle says, we cannot say that it has been happy, as no one can predict what new experiences will be confronted and how we will react. Life is not usually smooth sailing, and we can encounter many challenges and setbacks, so that even in old age we can suffer great misfortune. The loss of a child, serious illness, financial ruin and other vicissitudes of life can cause great unhappiness, and whatever success someone might enjoy, all of these misfortunes can occur in a life. If happiness consisted in the absence of misfortune, we could not call persons who have suffered tragedy fortunate or happy. Human beings, however, can overcome great tragedies, and Aristotle says that happiness does not depend on the fortunes of life, although good luck can make life more enjoyable. The happy person is someone who is happy throughout their life, because they spend their time in virtuous conduct and reflection, enabling them to bear whatever happens in the finest spirit. That is, the virtuous person is able to handle tragedy far better than someone who does not possess virtue. Aristotle (1976) defines the happy individual as the person who actively lives a completely virtuous life and who has enough material goods to provide for the basic necessities of life. Aristotle is mindful that human beings need to have their material needs adequately satisfied.

Happiness, as Aristotle understands it, is not merely connected to life's fortunes, but is the end result of possessing virtue. Aquinas comments that there are many goods that can be pursued – the good of health and that of fortune, for example – but all of these various goods are directed to one over-arching end, which is the ultimate good. He explains that Aristotle proposes that this ultimate good must meet two conditions: it must be perfect, and it must be good in itself – that is, not desired for something further. It is perfect because if it were not, there would be a further ultimate good that was perfect, and since it is perfect, it is desired for itself. This is because it is not something that only one person desires, but everyone. Aquinas (1993) notes that Aristotle only investigates the kind of happiness that is attainable in this life, and not what it might be for a future life, remarking that this is beyond the investigation of reason. For Aquinas, there is also a supernatural end for human beings, and this is to be with God. This is a gratuitous gift from God, and is a supernatural kind of happiness that goes beyond what is possible in this world.

The virtues in Aristotle

Having argued that happiness is the end of human beings and this is to be attained through the practice of virtue, Aristotle says that we now need to discover what virtue is and he begins consideration of this question by reflecting that the soul of the person is composed of two parts – a rational and an irrational part, the latter dividing into two, one which all living things share, namely, a nutritive part and another, which is an appetitive part which often strains against the dictates of reason, but in the sober or continent individual, can be brought under its control.[2] Virtue, too, is divided into classes in accordance with these divisions of the soul. Wisdom, understanding and prudence are intellectual virtues, whereas liberality and temperance are moral virtues. It is the intellectual virtues which enable us to know the truth and it is the moral virtues, the dispositions of our emotions, which enable us to respond to practical situations in the right sort of way. More generally, it is those states of persons which are praiseworthy which we call virtues. What is also salient here is that Aristotle understands – as do all virtue ethicists – that moral action cannot ignore human emotion. Human beings are not only capable of rational thought, but also of feeling emotion. Both elements are involved in deciding what moral action to take.

The virtues are to be understood as dispositions that contribute to the development of an excellent character, which is what enables human beings to attain happiness. There are different lists of virtues that can be compiled, but all of them will contribute in some way to the development of good character. Aristotle (1976) discusses the cardinal virtues of courage, temperance, justice and practical wisdom, but does not specifically name them as such, including only the first two in a list of virtues such as liberality, magnificence, magnanimity, patience, truthfulness and friendliness. Liberality, for example – the right attitude to money – has a prominent place in Aristotle's list of virtues. Aquinas (1981), in his adaptation of Aristotle, lists the cardinal virtues as the principal virtues, and develops a detailed list of secondary virtues, which include such virtues as *euboulia* (deliberating well), filial piety, perseverance, modesty, abstinence and sobriety, among others. In Confucian philosophy, the four main virtues are benevolence (仁, rén), dutifulness (rightness) (義, yì), propriety (rites) (礼, lǐ) and wisdom (智, zhì). There are also a number of secondary virtues (Shun, 2002). We have also mentioned such virtues as compassion, honesty, conscientiousness, care, integrity and respectfulness, which are more modern conceptions of virtues. Though these lists of virtues differ, they are all directed towards the task of the development of excellence of character, so that human beings attain their final end of happiness. We restrict ourselves to a brief consideration of the cardinal virtues.

The virtues do not simply exist in us, but must be brought into being in the same way that we acquire skills and capabilities in other walks of life. We do not become good builders without building things, or good players of musical instruments without playing instruments – nor, says Aristotle (1976), do we become morally good without exercising the moral virtues. We are constituted to acquire the moral virtues, but we do not have them without becoming habituated to their use. What makes just persons is their perform-ance of just acts; we become temperate by performing temperate acts and brave by performing brave acts. This makes sense, since we know that if we want to improve our ability to do something, we need to practise. A nurse needs to practise inserting a cannula into a vein if she is to become adept at doing it without causing the patient inordinate pain because she cannot find the vein. Similarly, if we want to be compassionate and kind in our dealings with patients, we have to practise compassionate and kind acts.

Aristotle (1976) regards practical wisdom as crucial in enabling us to determine what is the highest good for human beings. Aquinas also regards practical wisdom as the most important of the cardinal virtues, since it is the virtue that coordinates the others. In the *Summa Theologica*, he deals with it first after discussing the theological virtues of faith, hope and charity (Aquinas, 1981). It includes the ability to reach the correct conclusion through excellent practical thinking (deliberation) from correct premises by means of correct inference, and involves being able to make a correct assessment of one's situation and to apply the right moral knowledge to it. If we were in possession of it, we would always be able to make the right decisions, so our lives would be successful and happy. The importance of practical wisdom can be illustrated by considering its relation to moral virtue. Suppose we are in a situation where we need to give help to someone. Having the right virtue tells us that we should help that person, but does not tell us how we should help them. Practical wisdom leads us to be able to determine what the right action is in the situation. It leads to the right application of the moral virtue. Thus, if someone is drowning and we know we cannot swim, then practical wisdom tells us that the best course of action may be to throw the person a rope, which will enable us to haul them in. Throwing ourselves into the water would be foolhardy, and might result in both of our lives being lost.

A cardinal rule in determining what right conduct is, says Aristotle, is to realise that moral qualities are destroyed by excess and deficiency, and preserved by finding a middle path between these two extremes. This is called the Doctrine of the Mean, and urges us to be moderate in all things, avoiding excess and deficiency. To illustrate what he means, Aristotle says that, just as eating and drinking to excess can be as injurious to health as not eating or drinking enough, so too with the virtues. A person who shuns and fears everything and stands up for nothing becomes a coward, whereas a person who has no sense of danger becomes foolhardy. Likewise, a person who indulges in every pleasure and refrains from none becomes licentious, while one who shuns every pleasure becomes a bore (insensible) (Aristotle, 1976). Aristotle does not mean that we should just simply take a middle course in all cases, for sometimes the mean will be closer to one end than to the other. A virtue, he says, will nevertheless lie between the two extremes of excess and deficiency, both of which are vices. Rashness is an excess, and therefore a vice, because rash people are unable to assess the danger they face properly, and act without prudence, while cowardice is a deficiency, and therefore a vice, because cowardly people allow their fears and emotions to prevent them from doing what is right.

Aristotle emphasises the importance of schooling ourselves in the virtues: we do not just acquire them without effort. To become temperate, for example, we have to practise refraining from pleasures, so that when the time comes for us to have to actually resist indulging in pleasures (of a kind which would induce us to behave badly), we will be able to do so. This schooling, Aristotle agrees with Plato, should commence in infancy, so that the child is trained to feel joy and grief at the right things and to avoid the wrong things. If we have been correctly schooled, then we find acting virtuously enjoyable rather than irksome. Reflecting on the role that pleasure and pain play in affecting our behaviour, Aristotle says that it is obvious that virtue is also concerned with pleasure and pain. However, he does not mean this in a crude kind of way, in which what is right is determined by how we feel about it. It is clear that doing what is right and good can be pleasurable too, but it is also true that sometimes doing what is right and good can be difficult – hence the need to be properly schooled.

Doing what is right by itself is not enough, however, for just because someone performs a just action, this does not mean they are just – they also have to act in a certain way – to know what they are doing, to choose it for its own sake, and to do so with a fixed and permanent disposition, in other words, a disposition to act justly. For example, a person who acts justly by accident has performed a just act, but we would be unlikely to call them just as a result; or if someone acts temperately because they have run out whisky to drink, this is not going to count as being temperate. Something more is required, and this means not only knowing what the right values are and freely choosing them, but being properly schooled to be disposed to act in the right way. We must not only want to do the right thing, but must be disposed to do it as well. Virtue is the disposition that makes one a good person and causes one to perform one's function (as a human being) well (Aristotle, 1976).

There are three practical rules that can guide us in arriving at the mean between excess and deficiency, and so enable us to practise the virtues. First, we need to keep away from the extreme which is more clearly wrong than the other – that is, always aim to choose the lesser of two evils. Second, we must take note of our own inclinations (some things will give us greater pleasure than others) and drag ourselves in the opposite direction. Finally, we should guard against pleasure and pleasant things, see things for what they are and be impartial in our decision-making. In this way, we will be more likely to get close to the mean. No one, says Aristotle, is condemned for deviating a little from the mean; it is only those who go too far who are censured for their actions.

In his discussion of courage, Aristotle says that it is not just simply a matter of being between the extremes of fear and over-confidence, for there are some things that it is quite proper to fear – such as disgrace or harm to one's family. The courageous person will, however, be prepared to face the greatest of terrors. Yet there is a difficulty, for Aristotle warns that the courageous person will face fears in the right way and as principle directs, but will also fear the right things at the right time (Aristotle, 1976). The problem is being able to determine just what this means, for it is clear that there is a cognitive aspect to the exercise of the virtue of courage: we have to know how to act in the right way and at the right time. We have to be able to make the right judgements in relation to acting bravely and courageously. Courage is an important disposition to have when we are faced with a bad medical diagnosis or a prolonged treatment with an uncertain outcome. Aristotle notes that one of the greatest fears to be faced with courage is the fear of death. Similarly, knowing that the treatment we are about to undergo is painful and will lead to suffering also requires courage. The courageous person is prepared to bear pain, for this is much harder than abstaining from pleasure. However, it is not just bearing pain, for the courageous person is fully aware of what they face; it is also facing the mental pain and suffering that has to be borne.

Healthcare practitioners need to be sensitive to their patients, and to provide them with the appropriate support when they receive bad news. It is also the case that the healthcare practitioner needs to display a deal of courage in being able to convey bad news, both to patients and to their families.

In his consideration of the virtue of temperance, Aristotle returns to an earlier theme: the distinction between intellectual pleasures and bodily pleasures. He does not seem to think that there can be an excessive enjoyment of the pleasures of the mind, since intellectual pleasures are concerned with the love of learning, although he does say that there are those who like to pass their time listening to stories and spending their days in idle gossip. Temperance, though, is concerned with the pleasures of the body. He says that we do not call those with an excessive love of music, nor those who enjoy the smells of apples or roses, licentious, but we may well call people who enjoy the smell of food or perfumes licentious, for such smells remind them of the objects of their desires – in the first case, the gluttonous consumption of food, and in the latter, perhaps the arms of their lovers. For Aristotle (1976), the grossest pleasures belong to the senses of touch and taste. He notes that cases of deficiency in respect of pleasures scarcely exist, though clearly here we would want to include the ascetic, austere individual with a pathological hatred of anything pleasant. Aristotle regards the possibility of there being such an individual as remote, and believes that if there were such a person, they could scarcely be regarded as human.

Aristotle presents justice as a complete virtue because it is concerned with our relationship with others and requires us to exercise the other virtues if we are to act justly. It is the only virtue that secures advantage for another person and, when we act to do so, we are exercising the whole of virtue. Justice in that sense is not an individual virtue. When we think about justice in relation to the individual, Aristotle notes that we can understand being just as acting according to what is lawful and to what is fair. Aristotle discusses both distributive and retributive justice in terms of transactions between human beings. Where there are some goods to be distributed, this has to be done according to an agreed set of criteria. This means equal measures in the distribution are allocated to those adjudged equal according to the agreed criteria. Similarly, in the case of retributive justice, where a crime has been committed and someone has suffered an injustice, the judge has to attempt to restore equality (Aristotle, 1976). Justice as an individual virtue means that just individuals are those who are capable of choosing to do just acts, and this means in transactions ensuring an equal distribution. Just individuals do not act to advantage themselves above others. Importantly, Aristotle also acknowledges the centrality of our intentions in acting. That is, acting justly involves deliberation, and consciously choosing to act in a particular way. The person who, for example, returns a sum of money he has borrowed out of fear does not act justly. This is an important observation about virtues more generally, since it is not sufficient to simply exhibit virtuous behaviour, but to behave virtuously for the right reasons. This is because this is the kind of behaviour that is consonant with an excellent character.

Aquinas and the infused virtues

In his account of the virtues, Aquinas introduces the theological virtues of faith, hope and charity as being infused virtues. Aquinas (1981) agrees with Aristotle that the final end of human beings is happiness, but diverges from Aristotle by explicitly proposing that they also have a supernatural end, and that is to be with God. Through Christ, we are made participants in God's nature, so there is a supernatural happiness that transcends the worldly happiness that virtuous individuals can attain alone. Human beings, however, cannot attain this supernatural happiness without God's help, since it is beyond human power to do so. These virtues are called theological because their object is God, they are infused in us by God and they are made known to us through revelation in the scriptures. Aquinas says that human beings receive something additional from God in order for them to be directed towards their supernatural end. He says that first, in relation to the intellect, human beings receive certain supernatural principles that are held by means of a Divine light. These supernatural principles are articles of faith that are held through the infused virtue of faith. Second, the will is directed towards the supernatural end which, through hope, it is thought possible to attain. This hope is the infused virtue of hope. Third, through charity or love, the will is transformed by spiritual union with God – that is, through our virtuous actions, we draw ever closer to God until we are united with Him in love (Aquinas, 1981).

In a certain sense, all of the virtues come to us from God, since He is our Creator. (The seeds of the natural virtues are in us through possession of human nature. They have been implanted in us by God.) (Aquinas, 1998) They exist in us in potential, and need to be developed through practice. The infused virtues, however, are a different species of virtue because they are specifically ordered towards the supernatural end of human beings, which is God. The natural virtues enable us to achieve earthly happiness, while the infused virtues specifically direct us towards God. Our motivations for action in the latter case will be different. For example, a healthcare practitioner will act with compassion towards a suffering patient because this is what is required of someone with a compassionate character. and which is conducive to them becoming a fulfilled human person. The end they seek is their happiness. Someone who is moved to act in accordance with the infused virtues will act with compassion because this is required by the love of God, and so the action aims towards a supernatural end. Because human beings are free, the acts they choose will be meritorious if they are in accord with what is virtuous, and this means doing what is oriented towards the ultimate good, which is God. Our orientation towards God, however, cannot be reached through our own efforts, since this is a supernatural end, but is carried out through cooperation with God's grace (Aquinas, 1981). By acting in accord with God's grace, human beings can rightly hope that they will merit the reward of life with God. Through the action of charity – that is, God's love – the natural virtues can also be transformed into infused virtues, so that good actions, such as a courageous action, can also be done for the sake of the ultimate good.

Virtuous actions are performed because they lead to what is good for human beings, and for both Aristotle and Aquinas, this is happiness. They are not, however, performed for what they achieve for the individual. That is, they are not performed for the sake of the individual's happiness, but because it is a good action, and good actions – because they are good – lead to happiness. Aquinas holds that the ultimate end of human beings is to be with God, and this adds a further dimension to the moral actions we perform. To act virtuously is to act with love, since it is through charity, or love, that the acquired virtues themselves are transformed into infused virtues. This means that in our relations with other human beings, our moral actions must be motivated by love. For healthcare professionals, this means that in their dealings with patients, virtuous action is not just doing what accords with an excellence of character, but includes the added dimension of love of fellow human beings.

Reflective exercises

6.1   Can a person be virtuous and not happy? Review the discussion in this chapter on Aristotle's four cardinal virtues to respond to this question.

6.2 Only virtuous persons can act in truly caring ways. Present an argument that agrees or disagrees with this statement.

6.3 The virtues are acquired through habituation, according to both Aristotle and Aquinas. Most people, however, only rarely find themselves in hospital. How can they courageously face, say, a life-threatening operation if they have never practised doing so? Discuss how we might acquire the virtue of courage.

6.4 Prudence, or practical wisdom, is an important virtue to possess in the healthcare setting, as many decisions regarding treatment require discerning what is best for the patient. Is it just a matter of experience? Discuss how we might acquire the habit of practical wisdom.

6.5 Suppose an advocate of assisted suicide asserts that it takes great courage to decide to end one's life, and so is a virtuous action. How would Aristotle reply?

6.6 Aquinas argues that human beings have a supernatural end, so God has infused in them the theological virtues of faith, hope and charity. Suppose an atheist objects and says that he too can act from a love of his fellow human beings, so there can be secular versions of faith, hope and charity. Discuss.

6.7 Some contemporary secular philosophers such as Frenchman Andre Comte-Sponville argue that there are many more virtues than the traditional three theological and four cardinal virtues. Generosity, compassion and purity are three of the 18 virtues presented by Comte-Sponville. What do you think are the most important virtues for a health professional? Is it okay for some virtues not to be practised in the provision of healthcare?

6.8 Choose a mission statement from one of the Catholic Health Care organisations. Identify in these mission statements what virtues are presented as core to the purpose of the existence of the organisation.

Notes

1. Aristotle (1976) says 'Every art and every investigation, and similarly every action and pursuit, is considered to aim at some good.'

2. Alternatively, we can think of this second part as being part of the rational soul – in which case, says Aristotle, we can treat it as the immature or juvenile part of reason that has to be guided by the rational part of the soul in the proper sense.

References

Aquinas, T. (1981). *Summa Theologica,* trans. Dominican Fathers of the English Province. Westminster, MD: Christian Classics.

—— (1993). *Commentary on Aristotle's Nichomachean ethics,* trans. C. I. Litzinger. Notre Dame, IN: Dumb Ox Books.

—— (1998). *Disputed questions on virtue: Quaestio disputata de virtutibus in communi; Quaestio disputata de virtutibus cardinalibus,* trans. R. McInerny. South Bend, IN: St Augustine's Press.

Aristotle (1976). *Nichomachean ethics,* trans. J. A. K. Thompson. Harmondsworth: Penguin.

Australian Nursing and Midwifery Council (2008). *Code of professional conduct for nurses in Australia.* Melbourne: Nursing and Midwifery Board of Australia.

Oakley, J. (2013). Virtue ethics and bioethics. In D.C. Russell (ed.), *The Cambridge Companion to Virtue Ethics.* Cambridge: Cambridge University Press.

Oakley, J. & Cocking, D. (2001). *Virtue ethics and professional roles.* Cambridge: Cambridge University Press.

Shun, K. (2002). *Ren* and *li* in *The Analects.* In B. W. Van Norden (ed.), *Confucius and the Analects: New essays.* Oxford: Oxford University Press.

United Kingdom Nursing and Midwifery Council (2010). *Guidance on professional conduct for nursing and midwifery students.* London: Nursing and Midwifery Council.

7 Rationality in utilitarian thought

Jānis (John) Ozoliņš

Utilitarian thought in the Western world could be said to originate with Jeremy Bentham, an eighteenth-century philosopher and social reformer. Bentham introduced the principle of acting for the greatest good for the greatest number, which is at the heart of utilitarianism. Also known as consequentialism, utilitarianism has various forms, such as act and rule utilitarianism and preference utilitarianism. In its modern form, utilitarianism proposes that an action will be morally good if the good outcomes of the action outweigh the bad. This is irrespective of the nature of the action itself, so achieving the desired consequences is at the heart of judging the moral nature of the action. Its appeal is due to the conception of weighing up courses of action and deciding to pursue the one that results in the greatest benefits to all. However, it has its weaknesses, and these will also be considered in this chapter.

There is something appealingly intuitive about consequentialism and its offshoot, utilitarianism. Our daily lives are filled with choices, and unless we are prepared to simply act at random, in order to make the best choice we need to be able to evaluate them all. While in some cases there may be little to distinguish between choices, we normally try to choose the option that affords us most satisfaction. We choose a new car, a new phone or a new job by first working out a set of criteria that will help us to make up our minds and then by applying these to the available choices. For example, in buying a car we might compare different models on engine size, fuel economy, reliability and other relevant factors. In the end, our deliberations lead us to buy the particular car that best satisfies the set of criteria we have chosen. It would be odd if we chose a car we did not like or that we knew had major faults, such as bad brakes or poor steering. Our deliberation is directed towards weighing up our options in terms of good or optimal consequences. Similarly, when we are thinking about what we should choose to do in a particular situation, we choose what we think is the best choice, and this will be in terms of what we think the best outcome will be, all things considered. Consequentialism takes seriously the consequences of choosing a particular course of action. Weighing up courses of action, and deciding what to do in the hope of alleviating pain and suffering, is a staple requirement of healthcare practitioners, and consequentialism is beguilingly attractive. While consequentialism considers and assesses the consequences of an action, utilitarianism – an offshoot of consequentialism – tries to assess consequences in a more quantitative fashion.

In this chapter, we will begin with a brief account of classical utilitarianism, establishing the principle of utility, and the initial plausibility of the view that acting morally means bringing about the greatest good for the greatest number. Second, we will look at the difference between act utilitarianism and rule utilitarianism, two versions of utilitarianism emerging from classical utilitarianism. Third, we will consider some more recent developments of utilitarianism, such as R.M. Hare's (1952) preference utilitarianism and Singer's principle of equal consideration of interests. Finally, we will consider some objections to utilitarianism.

Classical utilitarianism

In Western philosophy, Jeremy Bentham (1907) is considered one of the early originators of utilitarianism, since he was one of the first to provide a developed account of the rightness or wrongness of an action based on the amount of pain or pleasure that it produces. Utilitarianism is a version of consequentialism, since it determines the rightness or wrongness of an action by a consideration of the results or outcomes of carrying it out. Consequentialism says that the rightness or wrongness of an action will be determined by how much good or evil flows from the outcomes or consequences of the action when it is carried out. For the consequentialist, the ends justify the means, which is opposite to a Kantian moral reasoning perspective. Consequentialism is a teleological theory, since it is concerned about ends rather than means. It is objective insofar as it takes into account all the interests of those affected by the proposed action. Bentham, and later John Stuart Mill (2009), believed that morality should be founded on objective principles – something that they did not think was the case with morality based on religious precepts.

Bentham (1907) begins from the postulate that human beings are fundamentally driven by pleasure and pain, saying that nature has placed man under two sovereign masters: pleasure and pain. The principle of utility, according to Bentham, is the principle of greatest happiness, by which he means the greatest happiness of all those with an interest in the action being contemplated. Furthermore, by happiness he means pleasure. The principle of utility, he explains, enables us to decide whether we approve or disapprove of an action in which we have an interest, according to whether it increases or decreases happiness. The principle can be applied to actions contemplated by private individuals or by governments. Utility, he continues, means that property in an object by which it produces benefit, advantage, pleasure, good or happiness (Bentham, 1907: 2). In other words, the best choice is the one that brings about the greatest good, not just from a personal point of view but from the view of all those who have a stake in the choice. Interests are to be considered objectively, not just from an individual perspective, and Bentham provides a hedonic or preference calculus for calculating the amount of pleasure or pain involved in a particular action. There are seven aspects to a pleasurable or painful experience: intensity, duration, certainty, nearness, fruitfulness, purity and extent. Taking these aspects into account, we sum up the values of the pleasures on one side and the values or disvalues of the pains on the other side, repeating the process for each person who has an interest in the proposed action. Putting these values all together, if we obtain a balance of pleasure over pain, the action is good, whereas if the balance of pain exceeds the pleasure then the action is evil. For Bentham, happiness equates to pleasure, so the greatest good will be brought about by the maximising of pleasure and the minimisation of pain.

Bentham reduces happiness and what is good to pleasure: it is the only thing that is self-evidently good in itself – that is, intrinsically good – while pain is the only thing that is self-evidently evil in itself – that is, intrinsically evil. This seems right, since human beings seek what they find pleasurable and avoid what they find painful. In addition, according to Bentham, human beings will choose what gives greater pleasure over what gives less pleasure. This, however, is problematic, since it makes no distinctions among pleasures. There is no distinction, for example, to be made between the pleasure of watching television all day and the pleasure of creating a new work of art.

John Stuart Mill (2009) was another early utilitarian. In his discussion of pleasure, he distinguishes between higher and lower pleasures, noting that it is better to be a human being who is dissatisfied than a pig who is satisfied, or Socrates dissatisfied than a fool satisfied. Mill notes that it is a mistake to suppose that pleasure for human beings is the same as that for animals – although it is true, since they are sensate like human beings, that they will feel pleasure and pain. Human beings have an intellect that makes them aware that happiness is more than the gratification of the senses. Mill says that mental pleasures are superior to bodily pleasures, and this is supported by the observation that where individuals are acquainted with both, they have a preference for a way of life that employs their higher faculties. Thus, for Mill, aesthetic and intellectual pastimes, and an interest in science and learning, are superior to bodily pleasures such as eating, drinking, having sex and being entertained. While it is possible that some human beings would be satisfied with indulging in bodily pleasures, Mill claims it is not just a matter of the quantity of pleasure, but also its quality that is important. The higher intellectual pleasures are of a superior quality because they appeal to those qualities of human beings that distinguish them from non-human animals (Mill, 2009: 14–20). Mill's argument that higher pleasures are better than lower pleasures, or merely sensual pleasures, is based on an understanding of human beings as having a greater dignity than non-human animals because of the nobility of human nature. Human beings are capable of rational and intellectual thought, of having the desire for liberty and to be moved by the love of others. He argues that it is not mere pleasure in the sense of bodily gratification that constitutes the good for human beings, but rather happiness, where this involves such things as close friendships, and appreciation of culture, beauty and truth.

Mill (2009) restates the principle of utility, or what he also terms the *greatest happiness principle*, to emphasise that it is not just pleasure that is to be pursued and pain that should be avoided, but what leads to happiness, understood to include the higher level interests and desires of human beings. Actions will be right to the extent that they produce happiness and wrong to the extent that they produce unhappiness. Although Mill retains the basic idea that utility is to be judged according to how much pleasure or pain is produced by a contemplated action, he broadens the idea of interests that need to be considered in determining whether an act is good or evil to include much wider interests. Hence it is possible to include higher level goals, such as health, in calculating whether or not a particular action should be under-taken. For example, someone may be suffering from tooth decay, and in order to deal with this, they will need to go to the dentist and face the pain of the needle and possibly of the extraction of the rotten tooth. Here the infliction of pain is necessary in order to accomplish a restoration of health, which is a good valued more highly than the infliction of pain during and after the extraction.

It is also evident that human beings are not, on the whole, satisfied by pleasure alone, and are capable of forgoing it in pursuit of other long-term goals. Mill warns, however, that human beings are also quite capable of forgetting that there are higher goals in life that will lead to a more fulfilling and lasting happiness, and tend to pursue sensual pleasures alone. For Mill, this is degradation, and arguably contrary to what is good for human beings. Mill notes that it is not necessarily the happiness of the individual that is important in utilitarianism, but the greatest happiness overall. As a result, he concludes that the cultivation of a noble character, whether or not it makes the individual happy, certainly makes those with whom such an individual interacts happier. Consequently, utilitarianism cannot attain its end of maximising overall happiness without the general cultivation of good character – that is without the cultivation of virtue.

Mill understands happiness to be no mere sensory pleasure, since it is momentary and lasts – perhaps intensely – for only a brief time; such pleasure is never permanent. Happiness is rather a life that includes such moments of pleasure, with few and transitory experiences of pain; with a variety of pleasures of different kinds, of activities rather than inaction, and contentment with what life is capable of granting, rather than dissatisfaction with what we have. Mill acknowledges that life will also include periods of pain and suffering, but happiness is the sum of all the experiences that a human being has, and not merely those at a particular point.

The key elements of utilitarianism

Emerging from our discussion of classical utilitarianism, the following are its key elements:

- It is a teleological theory, because happiness is proposed as the end of human activity.
- Happiness at its most basic is pleasure, but Mill points to a more sophisticated and nuanced understanding of happiness as being about human fulfilment.
- On the basis of observation of human behaviour, happiness is good.

- Because it concentrates on ends rather than means, it proposes that what is morally good is doing that which will bring about the greatest amount of good and least harm. The right action will therefore be one that produces more overall good.
- In determining what will bring about the greatest good and the least harm, we need to consider four questions:
  - What is to be understood by interests, desires and preferences?
  - How are we to determine the consequences of proposed actions (this is because utilitarianism is a species of consequentialism and is concerned with ends – we ask what the ends or outcomes are that we can foresee will occur if we act in a certain way)?
  - How are we to evaluate the foreseen consequences in terms of their good and their harm, based on the interests of all those with a stake in the proposed action, so that we can determine which action leads to the greatest good or greatest utility?
  - Are we prepared to accept responsibility for all the foreseen consequences of our action?
- Interests and desires can be understood in two different ways. They can mean either:
  - what we want and have a desire for, or
  - what is in our interest – not just what we want, but what is objectively good for us. Mill alludes to this in his discussion of what is good for human beings.

The key elements of classical utilitarianism appear in different forms in all theories of utilitarianism, clarified or modified in response to objections and problems to the theory. Some of these have already been indicated. For example, it is evident that pleasure and pain are not all that motivates human beings to act. There are difficulties in assessing interests and desires – especially in a healthcare context. A patient may be willing to endure significant pain in order to remain relatively lucid and able to engage in conversation. For the medical team treating the patient, this could be a difficult tightrope to walk, providing sufficient medication to enable the patient to remain lucid, but at the same time providing enough pain relief to prevent other complications. There is also the difficulty of the ambiguity between what we desire or want, and what is good for us. We might want to receive painkillers to alleviate a particular pain, but too much reliance on painkillers can lead to addiction. As a result, it is in our interests not to rely heavily on painkillers, using them as sparingly as possible.

Act utilitarianism

Act utilitarianism is the view that the rightness or wrongness of an action depends only on the total goodness or badness of its consequences – that is, on the effect of the action on all human beings (Smart & Williams, 1973). This formulation suggests that we take into account the effect of an action on all human beings, and this is clearly too strong a requirement. An alternative formulation proposes that we consider an act right and good if its consequences are at least as good as any alternatives (Frey, 1999). In act utilitarianism, we focus on a particular action and assess its consequences. If, on balance, more good results than bad, then the action is the right action to perform. For Bentham, goodness and badness of consequences could be determined by the amount of pleasure and pain that they engendered for all those affected by the action. Mill, on the other hand, required a more complex assessment of consequences, since he introduced a division between higher and lower pleasures. G.E. Moore (1988) introduced a further complication, in which certain kinds of things – such as knowledge – had intrinsic worth, irrespective of whether they produced pleasurable states. Hence, in Moore's assessment of whether a particular action produced more good than evil consequences, if one of the consequences produced an increase in knowledge, then the moral nature of the action would be deemed good. This is a development of utilitarianism because it acknowledges that there are some things that are good or valuable in themselves, which human beings might pursue even if they are not related to pleasure or happiness in a direct way. All of these philosophers, however, agree that the rightness or wrongness of an action has to be judged by its consequences.

The act utilitarian has to make two evaluations. First, if there are several actions that they could carry out, they have to decide what the consequences of each of them are and evaluate these in terms of their goodness or badness. Second, they have to decide which of the actions turns out to be the best on the basis of these calculations. Suppose there are two actions, A and B, and it is possible to determine all their consequences. The first task is to assess the goodness or badness of the consequences for each of the actions A and B. Having done this, the act utilitarian must decide which of actions A or B to do (Smart & Williams, 1973). At first glance, this seems simple enough: they will choose the action that brings about the greater amount of good, as the principle of utility enjoins us to do. This is so if both actions A and B were themselves equal in terms of implementation. However, it is possible, that, while the act utilitarian could carry out both actions, A will lead to better consequences, but is more difficult to carry out; or the agent may face other limitations that may prevent them choosing action A. For example, suppose a healthcare team has to decide between two possible treatments. The first treatment involves surgery, while the second involves a regime of medication. Both have been shown to be efficacious in different circumstances. Here the team needs to evaluate all the possible consequences of surgery, as well as the possible side-effects of the medication. In the former, there is the possibility that the surgery could lead to unwanted complications, and in the latter, the combination of medication required might not be appropriate for the particular patient and could cause some unwanted serious reactions. Having evaluated the consequences of both possible treatments, the team needs to decide which of the two is, on balance, the better option.

The second evaluation is not as simple as it might seem. It is not just a matter of choosing the action that has better consequences overall. For instance, suppose the health team had promised a patient that they would abide by their wishes in deciding on a course of action and the patient, having been presented with the recommendation that the best option is surgery, refuses surgery for their ailment. The patient may have a number of reasons for this and even though the team agree that surgery is the best option, they also need to take the patient's wishes into account. In this instance, the team would not be able to proceed with surgery, even though this is the better option for the patient. This highlights one of the difficulties for utilitarianism: if, on an objective evaluation, one option – here, surgery – turns out to be much better for the patient than a pharmaceutical alternative, then the utilitarian principle of maximising the overall good appears to be violated. The patient's refusal to undergo surgery prevents the maximisation of the good as regards the patient's health outcome. This leaves us with a difficult ethical problem, since the only option, if the good is to be maximised, is to override the patient's wishes. One possible response to this could be to say that the team should have included among the consequences an assessment of the possibility that the patient would refuse surgery, but this is not a consequence of the surgery, so cannot be included. Certainly, in hindsight, perhaps the team should have sought out the patient's views about surgery before evaluating the two possible actions, since this would have saved them the trouble of having to carry out the exercise in the first place.

The factoring in of the patient's views about surgery would be odd, since our assessment of the goodness or badness of actions, and hence whether the actions are right or wrong, would appear to depend on how an individual feels about an action and not on an objective assessment of it in terms of the expertise of the health team in relation to a health matter. Utilitarianism requires an objective assessment of all interests involved, but these do not include particular biases. Recalling that what is assessed is what is in a person's interest, not what they might be interested in, the issue is serious. The same problem arises in relation to the refusal of some religious groups of blood transfusions on religious grounds, even though in a number of cases such a procedure will save a person's life. A further evaluation of the options themselves is required, which is a separate exercise from the assessment of the consequences of each of the options. The value of respecting the autonomy of an individual or a group to decide something overrides the objective assessment of what is the optimal action to carry out. This suggests that there are complexities in practical situations that act utilitarianism by itself cannot handle.

Rule utilitarianism

Broadly speaking, rule utilitarianism holds that we follow certain kinds of rules selected for their efficacy in promoting the greatest overall happiness or social well-being in the evaluation of actions. Another way of stating this is the following. An action is a right or optimal one if it is required by a rule that is itself a member of a set of rules that are held to be more likely to lead to the overall greater good of society than any other such set of rules. This version of utilitarianism has appeal, because act utilitarianism does not provide guidance about how we should evaluate consequences, whereas rule utilitarianism provides rules that can guide the evaluation process. Intuitively, rule utilitarianism has some appeal when it is observed that human society is only able to function properly because there are rules that smooth our daily lives. For example, there are road rules that guide us in ensuring, as far as possible, trouble-free motoring, and there are laws, by-laws, rules and regulations that govern our lives in many other areas. It seems reasonable that there should be rules that help to regulate our actions so that what we choose to do brings about the greatest amount of happiness or social well-being. Rule utilitarianism holds that there is a set of rules to be followed that will maximise the utility of our actions (Pojman & Feiser, 2012).

The appeal of rule utilitarianism lies in the recognition that it is very difficult to assess all the possible consequences of an action or actions and then decide which action to perform. The goodness or rightness of the action depends on making such an assessment, and so agents are required to assess all the consequences that they foresee as flowing from the action. The problem is that there will be limits to the consequences that can be foreseen. This means that there will be innumerable consequences that are not foreseen, but that could have a significant bearing on the act. The butterfly effect (Smith, 1990) – a popular name for the realisation in chaos theory that a small change in initial conditions can have large-scale effects – is suggestive of the problem of whether or not the utilitarian can be expected to take responsibility not only for foreseen consequences, but also for the unforeseen consequences of their acts. We are inclined to say that they should not be, but it creates some uncertainty about whether the calculation of the amount of good is in fact the greatest good. This raises the question of how far the utilitarian's responsibility for consequences extends. If an event is remote from the action, we need to determine the extent to which responsibility diminishes in proportion to the remoteness of the consequence. This is because the extent to which the predicted amount of good or harm associated with the consequences of the agent's action needs to be included in the assessment of the overall rightness or good of the action.

One result of this reasoning is that the utilitarian will reject the principle that we perform that act which leads to the maximisation of overall happiness. This is because it is practically impossible to determine what it is that will maximise overall happiness or the greatest good, if the agent is to be held responsible for assessing all the consequences of a particular action – foreseen and unforeseen. Even if we say the agent cannot be held responsible for unforeseen consequences, given the remoteness of some foreseen consequences, it is also unfair to attribute these to the action of the agent. This is because some of these consequences will have other causes, and the agent's action may only be an indirect, contributing cause. Furthermore, some consequences may only be possibilities, rather than certain consequences of the action, and this too complicates matters. For example, if patients with a particular medical problem are to be treated with a specific medication, although all of the side-effects of taking it are listed, it is not usually expected that all of them will occur for every patient. Here the estimate of the good relies on a balance of probabilities that most patients will not suffer side-effects – or, if they do, the harms of the side-effects are outweighed by the benefits of the medications. In any case, practical considerations will limit the extent to which such deliberation can be undertaken.

The rule utilitarian provides a means of escaping this problem. Since the utilitarian has a set of rules to follow that can be held to maximise utility, in deciding how to act, they apply the rules to the proposed action. In a reasonably sophisticated version of rule utilitarianism, there will be three levels of rules. On the first level will be reasonably specific rules, such as those drawn from the Judaeo-Christian decalogue: 'Don't kill innocent people', 'Don't commit adultery', 'Don't lie', 'Keep promises' and 'Don't steal'. On the second level will be rules that apply in cases where there are conflicts amongst the rules. For example, if the local mafia boss asks us for the whereabouts of someone we know, we could be justified in not giving him the information by appealing to a second-level rule, which states, 'Don't give information to those who are likely to use it to harm others' or 'Where rules conflict, do what will cause least harm'. In this case, not passing on the relevant information might be the best option. An over-arching third level rule returns us to the principle of act utilitarianism – namely, 'If no other rule or set of rules applies, act in such a way as to bring about the greatest utility' (Pojman & Feiser, 2012: 106–7).

At first glance, it appears rule utilitarianism is a better option than act utilitarianism, because it provides us with guidance in the form of rules that have been accepted as moral norms that are taken to optimise the prospect of maximising the good. Moreover, where rules at the basic level come in conflict, there are second-order rules to help resolve the conflict. Finally, in cases where it is unclear how to proceed, there is an over-arching third-order rule, which is the principle of act utilitarianism. There are several problems that rule utilitarianism faces, and we will mention just a few. First, if the third order of rules returns us to act utilitarianism, there is the problem of preventing a collapse of rule utilitarianism into act utilitarianism. This alerts us to the fact that decisions about actions need to be made about particular cases; although rules provide guidance, they sometimes cannot be applied easily. This, in turn, leads to the conclusion that we have to consider each case individually, and so we are back with act utilitarianism. Second, there is the question of determining which set of rules can be claimed to be the optimal in generating the greatest amount of good. Not everyone will subscribe to the Judaeo-Christian decalogue, for example. Despite the biblical injunction against infidelity, some might believe that if two people are in love, they have every right to be together – even if they happen to be married to others at the time. Third, there is the problem of gaining consensus about the set of rules chosen as leading to the greatest amount of good. Suppose, for example, a group of people adopts a rule that says, 'Don't tell lies to members of our community, but tell them to those outside it (since they are not truly human beings like us) if it brings greater good to our community'. Fourth, there is the question of whether we want people always to comply with the rules, irrespective of whether they believe them or not. This raises the spectre of weighting certain kinds of values, such as freedom and conscience, compared with obedience to the established rules or laws. For example, it is required by Victorian law for doctors to refer a woman for an abortion to another doctor, even though they may conscientiously object to abortion. The assumption is that for the greater good, compliance with the law is required.

Preference utilitarianism

In R.M. Hare's (1981) view, moral thinking about problems will be improved if we think rationally. In particular, Hare says that we can improve our thinking about moral problems if we understand them, and this will mean understanding the words in which the problem is posed. Moreover, the meanings of words will be either partly or wholly encompassed by their logical properties. Careful studies of words like 'ought' and 'must', which are used in moral discourse, are to be understood in terms of their logical properties (Hare, 1981). In proposing this, Hare seeks to combine Kant's appeal to reason as guiding our moral actions with utilitarianism – that is, with the preferences of the people who will be affected by the actions that we are contemplating. He believes that the formal principles of utilitarianism are very close to Kant's categorical imperative – namely, that we ought to act only on that rule which will become a universal law. Working out the preferences of people is an empirical task, but Hare believes that if we have a perfect command of these, and are armed with an understanding of the logical properties of the words used in moral language, there will be little disagreement about what the right action to perform in a given situation will be.

This leads Hare (1981) to assert that moral judgements are both prescriptive and universal. They are prescriptive – that is, judgements we are bound to follow – because our understanding of the meaning of the moral language allows no other way to interpret what we ought to do, and they are universal because, by virtue of their meanings, there is no room for any alternative way of thinking about them. This means that if we say, 'Doing x to Y is right and good', then we mean, 'We ought to do x to Y'. This is prescriptive, since it prescribes what we ought to do. Second, if we say, 'We ought to do x to Y', it means that, 'Anyone else in the same situation as us ought to do x to Y and that if we were Y, we would be willing for x to be done to us'. This is universal, since it is expected that everyone would be willing to do the same thing in the same situation.

Importantly, Hare's (1981) formulation means that, since our moral reasoning is to be impartial, the preferences of others are as important as our own in the determination of what actions we choose to carry out. This means that we have a method for determining the greatest good because we put ourselves in the place of others by adopting their preferences and assessing them impartially alongside those that are our own. This method provides also for universalisable judgements about moral actions – that is, in identical cases, the judgements to be made are identical. Hare explains that if he says that he ought to do a certain thing to a certain person, he is committed to the view that the very same thing ought to be done to him were he in exactly the other person's situation – which would include having the same personal character-istics and in particular the same motivational states. Hare (1981) emphasises that equal preferences count equally, whatever their content; this is because the only question the method allows him to ask is one about what can rationally and universally be prescribed, or what is preferred from an impartial standpoint, if we were fully informed and made no logical mistakes.

Hare adopts both act utilitarianism and rule utilitarianism in his formula-tion of preference utilitarianism, since he acknowledges that there are simple cases in which our intuitions about how we should act will suffice in deciding how we should act. That is, there is an intuitive level of moral thinking in which we can apply a simple principle, such as 'do not kill', which will guide us in our moral decision-making. These simple moral principles are the product of our upbringing and our past moral decision-making. This is a simple form of rule utilitarianism. The difficulty with these is that, even in simple cases, it is not at all clear that the same intuitive principle will apply in a new situation, and in cases of moral conflict, intuitions will not suffice. Hare also states that in order to deal with moral conflict, we need a second level of moral reasoning, which he terms the critical level of thinking. The critical level needs to be supported by a number of relatively simple rules, but also dispositions to act according to them. Therefore, there are what Hare terms *prima facie* principles that corre-spond with *prima facie* duties that correspond to universal principles supported by very firm dispositions and feelings (Hare, 1981: 38–40). Critical thinking, which is to be applied in cases of moral conflict, will involve linguistic intuitions only, and not moral intuitions. It involves making moral choices based on the constraints imposed by the logical properties of moral concepts and the non-moral facts, and nothing else. When faced with a moral conflict, the process we adopt is to exclude consideration of any individual involved by universalising the case, so that the judgement we make will be the same in similar situations, and whether or not we are in the place of others affected by the action. Hare says that, at the critical thinking level, we employ both act and rule utilitarianism, since in cases of conflict we need to specify the act to be done as precisely as possible, and then apply the critical principles – which is act utilitarianism, since we are dealing with a specific act. It is rule utilitarianism insofar as the critical thinker selects general *prima facie* principles for use at the intuitive level (Hare, 1981: 40–3).

Preference utilitarianism has several advantages over classical, act and rule utilitarianism. In relation to act and rule utilitarianism, it enables both to be combined in determining what is a good moral action. It respects the objective, impartial and universal character of morality, since it invites the agent to weigh up all preferences – including their own – without bias. Preferences are simply those things in which the agent is interested; there is no need to consider anything about whether or not they are intrinsically good. This is because, in comparing and weighing preferences, we treat our own preferences no differently from anyone else's by making their preferences our own.

Peter Singer's principle of the equal consideration of interests

Australian ethicist Peter Singer extends preference utilitarianism by claiming that, for those who will be affected by our actions, we should give equal weight in our moral deliberations to all those with like interests. He extends preference utilitarianism by claiming that all sentient beings – that is, creatures capable of feeling pleasure or pain – have interests. Singer says that the principle acts like a pair of scales, weighing interests impartially. True scales will tip towards the side where the interest is greater, or where several interests combine to outweigh several smaller interests, taking no account of whose interests they happen to be. This means that we relieve X's pain, not because it is good to relieve X from suffering pain, but because it is good to relieve pain (Singer, 2011).

In extending the weighing of interests or preferences to sentient beings, Singer says that, in some cases, the interests of a non-human animal might be weighted more than those of a human being. Significant for Singer is whether a creature is capable of suffering or of experiencing enjoyment or happiness. If it is not, then it has no interests to be taken into account in weighing interest (2011: 50–1).

In considering interests as being linked to suffering or happiness, Singer agrees that the suffering of a non-human animal will not weigh as much as that of a normal adult human being who is suffering the same pain, since the adult would understand and dread the pain they were suffering. He does, however, suggest that where the human being is severely intellectually disabled or an infant, they will not suffer the pain more than the non-human animal. Hence, he asks, if we are prepared to experiment on non-human animals, why not on the severely intellectually disabled or infants (2011: 52)? In Singer's view, the salient question to ask in relation to interests is, first, whether those to whom the interests belong are equal and, second, whether the interests themselves are equal. If the answer is no to the first question and yes to the second, the interests cannot be weighed equally. Similarly, if the answer is yes to the first question and no to the second, the interests are not weighed equally. Since a newborn infant or foetus is not deemed an equal being compared with a normal adult human being, their interests will not weigh equally. This is because newborns or foetuses are not consciously aware of their past or future. This means, for Singer, that in certain cases, a newborn infant can be killed (2011: 126). This is without doubt an abhorrent conclusion, since it flies in the face of our moral intuitions.

Problems for utilitarianism

Undoubtedly the biggest challenge the utilitarian faces is in determining what is meant by the greatest good. Despite the attempt in preference utilitarianism to combine a rationally objective assessment of preferences that weigh the individual's preferences alongside others, it is difficult to see how subjective assessment of preferences can be avoided. For example, supposing that a terminally ill patient – a long-time member of an assisted suicide group – gains access to a large dose of Nembutal (pentobarbital), enough to end their life. It is rather implausible to propose that the patient will weigh interests in a manner that is objective in deciding whether to end their life. Their previous beliefs about ending their life at a time of their own choosing will undoubtedly influence their decision, since their view about what is good decides the manner in which preferences are assessed.

Other difficulties for utilitarianism include the following:

- If intense pleasure could be prolonged through connection to an apparatus that produced it, the problem of whether we would be justified in seeking to be attached to it permanently would arise. More significantly, on the other side of the coin, utilitarianism suggests that, for many people who are living lives of permanent suffering, their lives are not worth living.

- It is not clear the concept of the greatest good for the greatest number is coherent, since there does not seem to be any easy way of deciding whether to give $1000 to one person, or to give $100 to ten people or $1 to 1000 people.

- It is not obvious that objectifying and universalising preferences will lead to what is morally good. There seems to be a moral difference between the agent considered as the decision-maker in terms of weighing interests and being considered as one of those affected by the decision. A sado-masochist deciding whether to inflict pain on someone might readily agree that they would be willing to trade places with the victim.

- There is a problem of whether deciding to act for the greatest good for the greatest number is necessarily just, since it allows that an innocent person can be killed, for example, if it enables a larger number of individuals to be saved.

- There is difficulty in deciding whether one interest or good is to be preferred over another. Interests can be diverse – hence the difficulty of weighing whether someone's good name is worth more than someone else's pain or distress. For example, how would we weigh the considerable anxiety caused in a number of patients against the reputation of their surgeon if it were revealed that the surgeon had made mistakes in the past?

In contemporary healthcare ethical reasoning within Western cultures, utilitarianism is the primary normative framework to guide decision-making. In resource allocation, end-of-life care (in particular, assisted suicide and euthanasia) and ethical issues in the care of the pregnant woman, utilitarianism's pleasure and pain and greater good for the greater number principles guide moral action at the bedside, in the health institution and at the government policy and law-making level. It is therefore essential for any healthcare ethics debate at the micro, median and macro levels to engage more than just a utilitarian normative framework and to appeal to other perspectives, such as virtue and deontological ethical reasoning, where the motivation and nature of the action are carefully analysed, irrespective of the consequences.

Reflective exercises

7.1 Review the different forms of utilitarianism presented in this chapter, and highlight the key differences in their moral reasoning frameworks.

7.2 Suppose you are part of a health professional team treating a terminally ill patient, and the consensus is that further treatment is futile and life support should be switched off. However, family members are not prepared to allow this, and propose further aggressive treatment that they have heard about on the internet. Discuss how a preference utilitarian might find the greatest good in this given scenario, and what might be a recommended course of action.

7.3 You are part of a heart transplant team and an organ becomes available. You have two patients who are compatible and who are both in desperate need of the transplant, but obviously only one can be saved. One patient is a world-famous surgeon and the other a homeless man who is an alcoholic. Discuss, as a utilitarian, how you would determine the greater good.

7.4 Routine DNA testing of one of your patients reveals that she is genetically predisposed to a rare form of cancer. She has three sisters, but your patient does not want to tell them about the diagnosis. How would you apply the principle of equal consideration of interests in deciding what to do?

7.5 After pre-natal testing, a young couple has just been told that their first unborn child has Trisomy 18, which is a chromosomal condition associated with abnormalities in many parts of the body. The couple struggles financially, and has little family support. Exploring the different options for the couple with this diagnosis, utilise utilitarian reasoning to determine the course of action the couple could take.

7.6 The quality-adjusted life year (QALY) is a measure of disease burden, including both the quality and the quantity of life lived. It is strongly utilitarian in its orientation. Undertake a literature search on QALY and resource allocation in healthcare. What groups are advantaged and disadvantaged by such a resource allocation system? How would a utilitarian morally justify such a resource-allocation system implemented in society?

References

Bentham, J. (1907). *An introduction to the principles of morals and legislation*. Oxford: Clarendon Press.

Frey, R. G. (1999). Act utilitarianism. In H. La Follette (ed.), *The Blackwell guide to ethical theory*. Oxford: Blackwell.

Hare, R. M. (1952). *The language of morals*. Oxford: Oxford University Press.

—— (1981). *Moral thinking: Its levels, methods and point*. Oxford: Oxford University Press.

Mill, J. S. (2009 [1879]). *Utilitarianism*. Auckland: The Floating Press.

Moore, G. E. (1988). *Principia ethica*. New York: Prometheus Books.

Pojman, L. & Feiser, J. (2012). *Ethics: Discovering right and wrong* (7th ed.). Boston, MA: Wadsworth.

Singer, P. (2011). *Practical ethics* (3rd ed.). Cambridge: Cambridge University Press.

Smart, J. J. C. & Williams, B. (1973). *Utilitarianism: For and against*. Cambridge: Cambridge University Press.

Smith, P. (1990). The butterfly effect. *Proceedings of the Aristotelian Society*, 91, 247–67.

8 Natural law and the sanctity of human life

Jānis (John) Ozoliņš

The concept of natural law has a venerable past in the Western world, having its beginnings in ancient Greece. For example, in the Theban plays, Sophocles illustrates how human actions have to conform to the laws governing human beings that have been ordained by the gods. Natural law theory holds that an understanding of human nature reveals that there are basic human goods, which all human beings need in order to flourish and be fulfilled. Although there are differing views about what is to be included in the list of basic human goods, the broadest list includes life, work and play, beauty, truth, friendship, self-integration, peace of conscience, marriage and religion. Natural law holds that these goods are incommensurable, and one cannot be preferred over another – although some goods may be dominant in particular lives. Crucially, whether some goods dominate or not, we need to share in all the goods to some extent. This leads to some potential problems in terms of ethical decision-making.

The idea of a law

The idea of the natural law is very broad, and not only encompasses views about natural science and the laws governing natural phenomena, but also extends across a number of disciplines, such as law, politics, theology and, of course, ethics. In some respects, all of these areas in the natural law tradition intersect with one another, and arguably the natural law that lies at the base of all of these disciplines is the same natural law. It is claimed that it is the natural law that justifies our intuitions about what is morally right. It is morally right to do our best to heal our patients, for example, because one of the basic human goods is life and health. It is one we all need to lead flourishing lives. We shall provide a brief account of what we might understand by a natural law or law of nature, and then outline how the idea can be applied to develop a normative ethical theory with universal application.

Despite the acceptance of the provisional nature of many laws in the natural sciences, the idea that there are fundamental laws of nature that all physical objects in the universe obey because that is how things are is a central tenet of belief in the natural sciences. It is what drives scientists to keep looking for better and better explanations – and so more refined and precise laws of nature. Thus, despite modern Einsteinian corrections, Newton's law of universal gravitation is taken to hold in all places across the universe, and it is assumed that all physical objects will obey the law. Scientists – including medical scientists – are more often than not scientific realists who hold that what they investigate is an objective world independent of human beings, and so laws of nature are about the governance of relations between objects in an objective, mind-independent world. The physician interpreting an x-ray is confident that what they are observing is something in the real world – namely in the patient's body. Though there may be some variations in interpretation, the physician would regard it as irrational to hold that the truth of what the x-ray reveals is just a matter of opinion. Evidence-based medicine is premised on the view that there is an orderly world governed by laws. There is no room for a post-modernist version of medical science.

Applied in the domain of the human sciences, the same thought has its parallels – namely the idea that there are laws of nature that govern the actions of human beings. This does not mean that there are no aspects of what it is to be a living organism that are not governed by laws of nature, nor that there are no psychological aspects of what it is to be a human being that are not governed by laws of nature, but rather that there are rules of nature that, when followed, enable human beings to flourish and lead fulfilled lives. Human beings, as Aristotle notes, are conscious, rational and capable of making free decisions; however, because of this – unlike physical objects and non-conscious organisms – they are not subject to invariant laws (Aristotle, 1976). That is, once we know the masses of two objects and their distance apart, we can calculate the gravitational force between them, but the same certitude does not apply to human beings. Human behaviour cannot be predicted from antecedent conditions and known variables in this way. This creates a problem, for although human beings have the capacity to make rational and free choices, this does not mean that they will inevitably make the right choices. There is plenty of room for fallibility.

Nevertheless, the early Greek playwrights like Sophocles, observing human behaviour, recognised that some human activities and choices led to human flourishing, while others led to lack of fulfilment and misery. As a consequence, it was postulated that there were laws that must guide human behaviour in order for human beings to avoid misery and misfortune. The Theban plays are called tragedies for good reason because the human participants in the plays – like Oedipus – unknowingly transgress the natural law, but are punished all the same. Antigone boldly acts against Creon's enactment of a law prohibiting the burial of her brother Polyneices by claiming that his law is not unwritten and immutable like those of the gods, which demand that she fulfil her duty of filial piety (Sophocles, 2005). Antigone is aware of the higher law that she must uphold, while Oedipus is unaware that he transgresses the natural law. While it might seem unfair to us that unwittingly breaking the law should result in tragedy, the salient point is that human flourishing and happiness are dependent on human beings acting in accord with their natures.

The challenge for any account of natural law, when applied to the actions of human beings, is to reconcile human freedom with the understanding of natural law as dictating, in a deterministic fashion, how particular physical entities will behave. That is, if there are objective moral laws to which human beings are subject, then there does not appear to be any room for human freedom, since – like physical objects subject to the laws of physics – moral laws will compel human beings to act according to them. Human experience does not bear this out, however, and this leads to two possible explanations: either our moral laws are too crude and we have yet to discover the right ones or, since human beings are conscious and capable of reason, their deliberative choices are oriented to an end that they judge is their good, and although the end is determined, the means by which this end is achieved are not. Accepting the first explanation means human actions are determined by as yet undiscovered moral laws, but this has the unwanted consequence of taking away any responsibility for human action from human actors. Whether I act well or act badly can be explained in terms of some kind of evolutionary biological process, and human freedom is reduced to complex biological feedback loops, which act in order to enhance the survival of human genes. The effect of this is a very much diminished conception of the freedom, and by association the dignity, of the human being. The second explanation, which is the starting point for Aquinas's account of the natural law, begins with an Aristotelian understanding of human beings as conscious, rational beings who are oriented towards the good. This is not a short-term good that Aristotle sees as the end of human beings, but an ultimate end: the attainment of the supreme good. For Aquinas, this supreme good is God, and so is a supernatural end.

The classical account of natural law developed by Aquinas begins from an understanding of the human person as a composite being with a body and soul. This means that human beings are not just physical beings, but also spiritual beings that transcend the physical world. Their ultimate end is to be united with God, the supreme good, so we have a particular human anthropology. Aquinas says that the natural law is imprinted in the human mind, although he acknowledges that, on account of some impediment, a person may not act according to the demands of the natural law (Aquinas, 1948). Moreover, he adds, the requirements of the natural law may not be self-evident to everyone. He affirms, however, that human beings act for what they apprehend is the good, so the first principle of the natural law is that the good is to be done and evil is to be avoided (Aquinas, 1948). A salient point is that Aquinas believes that all human beings share in a common human nature, so natural law principles apply to all peoples and in all times. This view is not restricted to Aristotle and Aquinas, but is also to be found in classical Confucian literature in the thought of Kongzi (Confucius), Mengzi (Mencius) and Xunzi.

Practical reasoning and objective human fulfilment

Aquinas's natural law theory (NLT) is to be understood in terms of his observations of human behaviour. If we are to know anything about human nature, then the most sensible approach, according to Aquinas, is to see how human beings behave, and how they use their senses. He concludes that human beings are much the same everywhere, and so there is a common human nature that all share. Aquinas holds that neither skin colour nor gender indicates relevant differences when it comes to what is essential to human nature. Importantly, however, if we are to develop a normative ethical theory, we need to focus on the behaviours and actions of normal, mature human beings, ignoring secondary characteristics such as those mentioned. What distinguishes human beings from other animals is the capacity for abstract critical thought through the use of language and the capacity to make free choices. That is, human beings have intelligence, which is the capacity for rational thought and, crucially, free will. Human beings make choices, but these are not random: they are based on our needs and interests. More importantly, our needs and interests are directed towards a goal, one that all human beings share: the pursuit of happiness. This is the same goal identified by the virtue ethicist.

For Aquinas, as we have already said, this will ultimately mean being united with God. The difficulty is in being able to choose those actions that will lead us to happiness, which is what is good for human beings, since it is our experience that what we choose is not always what is ultimately good for us. Fortunately, we can know through critical reflection on human nature and human experience what our fundamental needs are. Once we have identified these, we will have a good idea of what we need in order to flourish as human beings. This will be the same for everyone.

The basic elements of what is good for us are not so hard to discover. In the natural world, we observe that plants need sunlight, water and soil in which to grow, and animals need food and shelter. They may also need the company of others of their kind, especially if the species is to be propagated. Different animals will also exhibit different degrees of consciousness, and will be able to experience pleasure and pain. They will avoid pain and prefer pleasure – a fact on which another universal theory of ethics, consequentialism, builds its account of ethics. Observing human beings, we know that we need the basics of food, clothing, shelter and security. Because we are aware that we are social beings, we know that we need the company of others, in friendship, but also in the organisation of a community and the state. This is because it is through coming together in community that we are able to develop fully as human beings. Finally, because we are reflective creatures, we need to discover knowledge and truth.

It is important to note that natural law theory does not begin with what is natural for human beings if that means just what we happen to be inclined to do or want. It is not necessarily the case that what is natural is good. For example, it may be natural for us to desire a life of comfort and ease, but it may not be good for us, as it may result in us failing to develop our talents as our comfortable life dulls our ambition to fulfil ourselves. It is natural to be inclined to consume foods we like, but they may not be good for us, as eating too much can lead to obesity and other illnesses. We may have to undergo an unpleasant cancer treatment that we would prefer to avoid, but it is necessary to preserve our life. There are numerous other examples. Classical natural law theory does not simply claim that what is natural is good; rather, it begins with what human beings need in the sense of what is objectively good for them. Thus what we think is good for us may turn out to be not what is really good for us in terms of reaching our ultimate goal of happiness.

Our natural inclinations are therefore a useful guide to what is good for us, but they are not a trustworthy one, as following our natural inclinations, desires and wants will not always lead to our good. In order to discern whether a proposed action will contribute or lead to our good, we need to use practical reasoning. It is our ability to consistently, and to a certain extent spontaneously, make good decisions about what actions lead to our happiness (our ultimate good) that Aquinas recognises as the possession of virtue. It is not a matter of acting in accord with our particular natures, but in accord with what we might reasonably expect is our good.

Aquinas reflects that there is an order to our natural inclinations, and this serves as a guide to the order of the precepts of natural law. That is, there is a hierarchy to the basic human goods. First, he says that – like other living things – human beings seek to preserve their own lives, and will seek to do this by whatever means will achieve this. Though he does not specifically say so, we would include food, shelter and physical security as means of preserving life. Second, Aquinas says that we also need those things that we share in common with animals, such as sex, and the need to rear and educate our young. Third, as a result of possessing reason, human beings have an inclination to know the truth about God and to live in society, to shun ignorance and to avoid offending those others with whom we have to live (Aquinas, 1948). The hierarchy he provides is anticipatory of Maslow's (1943) hierarchy of needs, where basic physical needs are at the bottom and higher level needs are at the top. He does not elaborate further, but in all of these, human beings are guided by the unifying principle of natural law, which is a law of reason – namely, that human beings are to act so that good is to be done and evil avoided.

Contemporary natural law theory

Contemporary natural law theory has sought to elaborate the natural law theory enunciated by Aquinas, but also to move beyond it. Although there are some differences among those who have developed contemporary natural law, they take as their starting point Aquinas's enunciation of the first principle of natural law, together with his observation that this principle is known self-evidently through practical reason – that is, it is obvious that human beings will want to do what they apprehend is good and avoid what they think is evil. This leads him to conclude that all the natural law precepts based on this first principle – since they are also known through practical reason – are also self-evident. In contemporary natural law, these natural law precepts are called basic human goods, and are held to be self-evident, irreducible goods that human beings need in order to be fulfilled.

According to contemporary natural theorists Grisez (1983) and Finnis (1980), human well-being and fulfilment are constituted by basic human goods. Finnis initially identifies seven basic goods: life, knowledge, play, aesthetic experience, sociability or friendship, practical reasonableness and religion. Grisez agrees that life is a basic human good, as are knowledge and truth, practical reasonableness, sociability or friendship, religion, play and skilful performances, which enable sharing in culture. This can be regarded as aesthetic experience. Grisez, however, builds on this work of Finnis, identifying harmony as a characteristic of several of the basic human goods. Harmony has two aspects: one in which we are in harmony with others (friendship and sociability) and the other in which we are in harmony with ourselves.

Four of the basic human goods, says Grisez (1983), can be called reflexive goods, since they are both reasons for choosing and are in part defined in terms of choosing. The reflexive goods are self-integration, which is harmony among all the parts of a person which can be engaged in freely chosen action; practical reasonableness or authenticity, which is harmony among moral reflection, free choices and their execution; justice and friendship, which are aspects of human sociability and capacity to act in harmony with one another; and religion, which is harmony with God. These reflexive goods, according to Grisez, are moral goods, since they fulfil human beings in the existential dimension of their being. By this, we take him to mean that these goods are necessary for us to be able to realise ourselves as human beings or live as human beings, since they require us to act. That is, we cannot be fulfilled by the good of friendship unless we choose to be a friend to someone.

The substantive goods are: life itself, including health, physical integrity, safety and sex; knowledge of truth and appreciation of various forms of beauty or excellence; and activities of work and of play (Grisez, 1983). Later in his further exploration of the basic human goods, Grisez also identifies marriage, the fruitful and intimate union between man and woman, as a basic human good. Practical reasonableness has two aspects: harmony among judgements, choices and performances; and harmony among one's moral choices, which is identified as peace of conscience. It should be noted that peace of conscience is not a moral good, but rather a basic human good. With this addition, the number of basic human goods comes to nine. There are undoubtedly other ways in which we might divide the basic human goods. The salient point, however, is not how many basic human goods there are, but that there are basic goods that contribute to our fulfilment as human persons. They are intelligible as basic goods that contribute to our well-being.

Grisez, in describing the basic human goods, compares them with their opposites. Beginning with the substantive goods, their basic nature can be seen through contrasting them with evils, understood as privations or the absence of human fulfilment. Thus death, sickness, infertility and lack of shelter or security are contrasted with the good of life, which includes health, shelter and security. The vast effort to provide healthcare is premised on the need to alleviate the evils of disease and illness. Second, we can contrast the evils of hard, monotonous and unremitting work or of unemployment with skilled performance, as well as the good of play and recreation. Boring, monotonous work is unfulfilling, and we can see that what is missing is the basic human good of being able to use one's talents in creative activity that is personally satisfying. Third, the evils of ignorance and falsehood point to our need for the basic good of knowledge and truth. Fourth, ugliness and disorder are contrasted with beauty and aesthetic experience. The experience of living in an environment that is marred by ugly, defaced concrete buildings and surrounded by rubbish is soul destroying, whereas that of living in an environment in which attention has been paid to the aesthetical design of buildings and in which beauty is preserved will undoubtedly lift the human spirit and enable people to enjoy life.

Similar contrasts can be found for the reflexive goods. Anxiety, loss of self-control and insanity are evils, and are contrasted with the good of self-integration, the harmony between feelings, choices, judgements and actions. Here the evil is not leading a chaotic, bohemian life – which someone might prefer; rather, it is leading a life in which there is a loss of control over one's life because of an inability to make judgements or choices. Feelings of guilt and self-hatred can be contrasted with the second reflexive basic human good of peace of conscience, which involves harmony among our moral judgements, actions and choices. Here the evil is a self-loathing and lack of self-respect brought about by dissatisfaction with one's life because of the moral choices that have been made. Loneliness, hostility and war are the evils that result from the lack of the third reflexive good of friendship, which includes harmony between people. While it is true that some people prefer their own company, and so will not feel lonely, nevertheless none would welcome others to show open hostility that leads to harm being done to them. The evil of impersonal and anti-social sexual activity can be contrasted to the good of marriage. Sexuality and sexual activity is a basic human good, as we have already said, since it has a natural biological activity that we share with animals: the aim of procreation. In that sense, it is a basic good. Human relationships are more complex, however and, just as we recognise the good of friendship, the good of marriage is the development of a deep, intimate and harmonious relationship between a man and woman, which encompasses sexual intimacy, having children and their nurturing within that loving relationship. The evil, in contrast, is the use of other people not just for sexual gratification, but for shallow, temporary relationships that demand little commitment or involvement with the other. The final reflexive good can be contrasted with the evil of alienation from God. Here it is not just a matter of religious belief for, as we know, there are many who do not believe in God. We can understand the evil here as an alienation from a sense that there is something greater than us to which we can be committed. Without such a sense, we may become self-centred and selfish. The basic good of religion is harmony with the sacred, with what is part of the mystery of life and of our existence.

In summary, we can say that the first four goods – the *substantive goods* – do not depend on our self-conscious choice: we are all able to participate in them without being aware of it. However, the next five goods – the *reflexive goods* – are forms of harmony that require our self-conscious experience and choice. Pleasure is not one of the basic human goods because it appeals directly to our senses, whereas the basic human goods are intelligible, and provide the reasons for our actions and choices. Pleasure is just feeling. Pleasure is only good when it is the pleasure associated with the pursuit of a basic human good, such as the pleasure of friendship. The basic goods are personal, communal and open-ended. This is because participating in them enables us to live more fully, to be fulfilled persons. All of the basic human goods are equally basic: none can be regarded as superior to any other, though we can divide them into substantive and reflexive goods, as well as propose a hierarchy, which simply reflects the thought that if we do not have life, none of the other basic goods can be pursued. Because the basic goods cannot be weighed against each other, they are incommensurable – that is, we cannot favour one basic good over another. As we have seen in classical natural law theory, the basic moral norm that we do good and avoid evil demands that we respect each of the basic human goods. Grisez (1983: 184) restates the fundamental or basic moral norm in the following way: 'In voluntarily acting for human goods and avoiding what is opposed to them, one ought to choose and otherwise will [choose] those and only those possibilities whose willing is compatible with a will to integral human fulfillment.' Thus we should respect our own well-being and the well-being of others in all our choices and actions. Natural law theory aims for the good, considered as the fulfilment of each individual.

From the basic moral norm and the basic human goods, it is possible to begin to develop specific moral norms that respect or uphold the basic human goods. Thus we will specify particular moral rules such as 'don't lie', 'don't steal', 'don't cheat' and so on, which respect the basic human goods, such as truth, sociability or friendship, and peace of conscience. In order to develop moral rules to guide our actions, Grisez (1983) develops what he terms the modes of responsibility and connects them to the virtues.

Modes of responsibility and the virtues

The modes of responsibility enable us to connect to the qualities that we require in order to be able to pursue the basic human goods that will lead to our fulfilment. We need, for example, various virtues to help achieve our goals. We need fortitude or courage if we are to overcome the obstacles and hardships that we might encounter in our lives; we need temperance to moderate not only our desires, but also sometimes our ambitions. We need to deal with others and ourselves fairly, and so we will need to exhibit justice. The connection between natural law theory and the virtues is close, since not only do the virtues lead us to do what is right, but also to develop our moral characters. Since natural law is concerned with the nature of human fulfilment and the pursuit of happiness, it is also concerned with the pursuit of the virtues, because these are directed to the achievement of these ends. The virtues embody the modes of responsibility (Grisez, 1983).

Virtue in natural law theory – as in virtue ethics – is a disposition to choose to act and live in a manner that leads to the good, for oneself and for others. It means acting in a way that respects the basic human goods. Vice, on the other hand, is the opposite: a vicious person chooses to act and live in a manner that deliberately damages one or more of the basic human goods. For example, someone who shows little regard for their health by engaging in the taking of recreational drugs and promiscuous sexual activity damages a basic human good. A vicious person does not respect others, and if they are a manager or an employer, for example, will treat their staff with contempt, subject them to poor working conditions and exploit them as much as possible. The modes of responsibility provide a framework for specifying the virtues, but also vices. Grisez (1983: 205–22) lists eight modes of responsibility, which he claims correspond to the eight beatitudes:

- *Preparedness to act.* One should not be deterred by felt inertia from acting for intelligible goods. We should not be lazy.
- *Willingness to share.* We should not be pressed by enthusiasm to act individualistically for intelligible goods.
- *Possession of self-control.* We should only act to satisfy an emotional desire if it enables us to attain an intelligible good. That is, don't just act to satisfy emotional cravings.
- *Courageousness.* We should not be afraid to act because of fear of pain, or repugnance or fear of some other obstacle.
- *Fairness.* We should act impartially when our acting affects other people. We should not let our decision-making be shaped by our likes and dislikes, but by the intelligible goods for which we aim.
- *Sincerity or clear-headedness.* We should act soberly according to the reality of a situation, and not delude ourselves through emotion or rationalisation into distorting our perception of what we are doing.
- *Forebearance.* We should always reject any feelings of hostility or resentment towards the basic human goods, and avoid any damage to them.
- *Respectfulness towards all the basic human goods.* We should avoid damaging one basic human good in the pursuit of another. We should not attempt to weigh or measure one good against another.

Absolute moral norms

Although some moral norms are non-absolute, because they are open to further specification, there are some that derive from the modes of responsibility – especially the final one, respectfulness towards all the basic human goods – that are absolute or exceptionalness moral norms. For example, it is wrong to kill innocent human beings, it is wrong to rape, it is wrong to deliberately destroy another person's sanity or identity, and it is wrong to commit adultery. Any deliberate attempt to damage one of the basic goods in our own lives or in the lives of others is morally wrong in principle, no matter what good may be achieved or what harm avoided by that action – it is wrong, no matter what the consequences.

Because most moral norms are non-absolute, we need to use our reason in order to make judgements about how to act. There are many situations in our lives when it is difficult to decide how we ought to act. We first need to have a clear understanding of the situation in which we find ourselves, and to be able to discern, through making use of the modes of responsibility and without violating any of the basic human goods, how we should act. We are assisted in this by the connection between the modes of responsibility and the virtues. The modes of responsibility are a development of the classical or cardinal virtues: justice, courage, temperance and prudence (practical wisdom). The last of these, practical wisdom, is the central organising virtue in natural law theory, but we cannot have this virtue without having the other three. That is, we cannot develop prudence or practical wisdom without having developed the others. It is impossible to judge wisely if we lack courage or lack temperance to have the wisdom not to give in to temptation. Hence the virtues also form an integrated whole.

Moral absolutes and the double effect

A major problem faced by natural law theory – although all ethical theories face this – is dealing with moral dilemmas. For the natural law position, cases of genuine moral dilemmas are those in which there are clashes between incommensurable basic human goods or between incommensurable expressions of a basic human good. These appear to be irresolvable. For example, suppose a young pregnant woman has been admitted to hospital suffering from a rapidly metastasising cancer, which is threatening to invade her placenta. Her pregnancy has reached 21 weeks but the treating clinicians have concluded that aggressive treatment of the cancer will result in the death of the child. Doing nothing, however, will result with certainty in the cancer spreading to the placenta within the next two weeks, and will bring about the death of the mother, as well as the child. Existing technology is unlikely to save the child. The young woman also has other young children. To save the woman, the only viable option is to deliver the child prematurely and treat her cancer, as delay will kill them both. Here the good of the life of the mother clashes with the good of the life of her child. If you deliver the child, it is certain it will die; if you do not, both will die. The dilemma for natural law is how to deal with the clash of incommensurable expressions of a basic human good or the clash between incommensurable basic human goods.

Natural law has strategies that enable it to deal with some cases in which resolution of the apparent incommensurability that involves the weighing of goods can be found. Some of these are listed below:

- Some cases will involve a moral norm which is not exceptionalness – that is, one that is not a moral absolute, such as keeping a promise. For example, a promise to buy someone's car might be voided on discovering that it was actually rusted through and the engine had seized up.
- Some situations may be resolved by further elaboration of the cases. Sartre (1975) gives the example of the young man who has to decide between remaining with his sick and elderly mother and looking after her, or joining the Resistance. This could be resolved by knowing the extent of the mother's infirmity, whether or not someone else could look after her, whether joining the Resistance would mean going to another part of the country and so on.
- Some cases could involve an attempt to minimise harm, since the problem itself cannot be solved. For example, providing safe injection rooms for drug addicts, while not condoning their activities, could be seen as seeking to minimise the risk to their health. This is a more difficult example, since it leaves their actual addiction problem untouched. Arguably, this could be said to violate some of the basic human goods. An example of the difficulties with this suggestion is supposing a father gives his daughter money to buy drugs rather than allow her to become a prostitute to get the money. Superficially, this looks like a form of harm-minimisation, but it violates several of the basic human goods.
- Some cases can be resolved by giving a more elaborated definition of the moral principle at stake. For example, lying could be defined as telling someone a falsehood with the intention to deceive, or telling someone with a right to the truth a falsehood with the intention to deceive. Thus the Nazis need not be told the truth about the whereabouts of a Jewish family someone is hiding. An objection here might be to ask who has the right to the truth – the Taliban would reject any suggestion that the United States has a right to know the whereabouts of an al-Qaeda terrorist.

A significant strategy in the armoury of natural law theory in dealing with moral dilemmas is the principle of double effect (PDE). The traditional formulation of the principle of double effect is that it is not morally permissible to choose and perform an evil act (that is, an act that involves the direct intention to damage one or more basic human goods) even though the act is a means to achieving some good or goods; however, it may be morally permissible to choose and perform a good act even though the act has a foreseen but unintended harmful effect under the following conditions:

- The act to be done must be good in itself.
- The good intended must not be obtained by means of the evil or harmful effect.
- The evil or harmful effect must not be intended for itself, but only permitted.
- The evil or harmful effect must not be disproportionate to the good intended.

Central to Grisez's analysis of double effect is the notion of the indivisibility of the act: there is equal immediacy of the good and bad effects. Thus one cannot commit an adulterous act to save one's children from the prison camp, since the saving effect is not present in the adulterous act, but rather in a subsequent act. He distinguishes between what one chooses to do and what one bears responsibility for as being foreseen side-effects. What one brings about is far more extensive than what one chooses to do. Thus someone who chooses to play their stereo at full volume at 3.00 am may intend to listen to music but, unless completely obtuse or living in an isolated part of the world, they should foresee that this would wake the neighbours and ruin their rest. A further foreseen result of this choice might be the ruination of the health of the neighbours and possibly a loss of their jobs. (Say, for example, they were all involved in highly dangerous occupations requiring an extraordinary degree of alertness.) Grisez (1983) echoes Aristotle by arguing that one determines oneself primarily in choosing particular courses of action, since it is these choices that establish the kind of person that one is becoming. He holds that one is secondarily responsible for the foreseen consequences of carrying out the acts one chooses. This means that it is important to ask whether one is prepared to accept these.

Recalling that Grisez's analysis of natural law theory involved the formulation of modes of responsibility in guiding our moral choices, the eighth mode of responsibility enjoins us not to damage or destroy one basic human good in the pursuit of another. This means that, in determining how to act, non-absolute norms yield to absolute norms – that is, we order our norms in such a way that where there is a clash between absolute norms and any others, we never choose to violate that which is an absolute. I may desire to live comfortably, but this does not mean that I can choose to rob and kill people to achieve this. Of more immediate interest to us, however, is the case where there is a clash between absolute norms. Though the eighth mode of responsibility precludes a choice to destroy, damage or impede a human good, it does not rule out accepting foreseen side-effects that it would be wrong to choose. Hence such side-effects may be accepted unless some other mode of responsibility requires the contrary. Grisez (1983: 298) says that

> therefore, the problem of when one may act in a way which one foresees will have humanly bad effects can be solved only by considering all of the intelligible features of that about which one is deliberating, referring to all the modes of responsibility, and articulating a norm for the act under consideration. The act will be right if and only if in choosing it one violates none of the modes of responsibility.

Grisez is saying that we cannot deliberately choose to damage, destroy or impede a human good, but this does not mean that we cannot permit the damage, destruction or impediment of a human good to take place.

This brings us back to the importance of proportionate reason, the fourth condition of double effect. In choosing to uphold the value of human life, do we permit, say, a friend to be betrayed, thus harming the good of friendship? Ordinarily, we would regard it as wrong to betray a friend. Suppose, however, that our best friend is a murderer, condemned to death, who escapes from prison and seeks refuge with us. There may be a variety of reasons why we should allow him shelter – for example, he may have saved us from drowning, prevented our sister from being raped and been a wonderful supportive friend before he became drug addicted and took to a life of crime. Should this friend now be betrayed to the authorities who have come searching for him? What if we are opposed to capital punishment? This would seem to be a case where we permit harm to the good of friendship in order to safeguard the lives of others – although of course here there is the further complication that we also harm the value of the individual human life of the murderer, since he will be returned to death row. The importance of proportionate reason for the act of betrayal – and so harming the good of friendship – is evident. If our friend really is a violent and dangerous murderer, then there is good reason to give him up to the authorities. Alternatively, we could argue that someone who is a dangerous and violent murderer has forfeited the usual obligations of friendship. Suppose that, instead of betraying a guilty, criminal friend, we betray an innocent friend because we are convinced that this would save the world from annihilation – would this count as a proportionate reason? The answer is no, since we are using an evil means to achieve a good end. In the previous case, though we were betraying our friend, the act could also be described as cooperating with the lawful authorities in apprehending a dangerous criminal. This act is not evil in itself. Socrates' injunction to us is plain: 'It is better to suffer evil than to do it.'

In the example of the pregnant mother, the criterion of proportionate reason would lead us to consider whether there is a proportionate reason to deliver the baby prematurely, knowing that it is almost certain that it will die, since the outer limit for survival with current technology is 23 weeks. The option of doing nothing because we do not want to violate the good of life results in both their deaths. Delivering the child to save the mother is a proportionate reason for acting, since it is the only action that can give the mother a chance of surviving. Moreover, if the evil act – presiding over the child's death – is foreseen but not intended, and it occurs at the same time as the good act of saving the mother, which is intended, then according to natural law, we are justified in acting.

The intention that we have for acting is important. In discussing an analysis of Aquinas's argument about how we should respond when someone physically attacks us, Grisez (1983) acknowledges that an unborn child is not an unjust aggressor, but argues that there is no choice but to kill. The morality of what is done therefore depends upon fairness and other modes of responsibility. This echoes what Aquinas himself says. He notes that there is nothing that hinders the one act of self-defence having two effects: one the saving of one's life and the other the killing of an aggressor. The intention of the agent is important, but Aquinas also warns against carrying out an act that is out of proportion to the end. He says that while we are justified in acting to save our own lives, it is wrong to *intend* to kill another in self-defence; nor is it permitted to kill someone in one's own defence *out of spite*. Thus one is not given any licence by the principle of double effect to retaliate in a manner out of proportion to the attack.

Conclusion

The strength of natural law theory is that it provides a universal normative ethical theory based on the observation of human nature, and extracting from this an account of the moral principles that will enable human beings to live flourishing lives. Although there are some arguments about what constitute the basic human goods, it is difficult to deny that there are common basic needs that human beings require in order to both survive and to live fulfilled lives. Without the substantive goods, such as life and health, there is no possibility of human flourishing. Arguably, the reflexive goods, which recognise the need for human beings to be in harmony with themselves, with others and, for theists, with God, are also basic to human flourishing. Finally, natural law argues that there is an objective moral order, and that there is a fact of the matter about whether an action is morally right or wrong. That is, a statement that it is morally right to act in a particular way can be true or false.

This is not to say that there are no difficulties for natural law. The first is the question of what kind of law is a moral law, given that it is not the same as a physical law. The second is explaining the nature of human freedom and its relationship to natural law. A third is in the application of double effect in cases of moral dilemmas, where it may not be easy to determine whether or not we are acting proportionately.

Reflective exercises

8.1 Knowledge is one of the basic goods, but is it true that pursuing knowledge is always good? For example, is pursuing medical research that leads to the development of biological weapons good? Discuss.

8.2 Why isn't pleasure one of the basic human goods? Discuss.

8.3 What do we mean by human fulfilment and flourishing? Consider the case of a woman who gives up her highly successful career in order to care for her elderly mother, who has dementia, or the father who works part time in a low-paid job so that he can care for his daughter with a severe physical disability. Discuss.

8.4 Is proportionate reason just another way of weighing preferences? Discuss.

8.5 Suppose you are in charge of treating a terminally ill patient who is being fed through a percutaneous endoscopic gastronomy (PEG) feeding tube. The patient is increasingly failing to respond adequately to the regime of drugs she is taking, and the feeding tube is becoming distressing to her. She begs you to remove the tube and allow her to die. Discuss how natural law theory can help you decide what morally appropriate action should be taken.

References

Aquinas, T. (1948). *Summa theologica*, trans. Fathers of the English Dominican Province. New York: Benzinger Bros.

Aristotle (1976). *Nichomachean ethics*, trans. J. A. K. Thomson, rev. trans. H. Tredennick. Harmondsworth: Penguin.

Finnis, J. M. (1980). *Natural law and natural rights*. Oxford: Oxford University Press.

Grisez, G. (1983). *Christian moral principles: The way of the Lord Jesus (Vol. 1)*. Chicago: Franciscan Herald Press.

Maslow, A. H. (1943). A theory of human motivation. *Psychological Review*, 50(4): 370–96.

Sartre, J-P. (1975). Existentialism is a humanism. In W. Kaufman (ed.), *Existentialism from Dostoevsky to Sartre* (rev. and exp. ed.), trans. W. Kaufman. New York: New American Library.

Sophocles (2005). *Theban plays of Sophocles*, trans. D. R. Slavitt. New Haven, CT: Yale University Press.

9 Obligations, duties and rights

Jānis (John) Ozoliņš

In the last decade, there has been a resurgence of utilising a Kantian theoretical approach in healthcare ethical reasoning. Kant (1909, 1991, 1997) argues that morality does not depend on how one feels about a particular action, but rather on whether one approaches the action with a good will. Kant believes that the moral life is based purely and simply on duty or obligation, and not on a utilitarian calculation of the best consequences or on a natural law respect for the basic human goods. So Kant holds a *deontological* view of ethics – an ethics of duty or obligation. Kant says that the most important thing is to will to do what is rational to do, and what reason commands. He says that the principle according to which we should act is to do what we would want to be a universal law – that is, we would want everyone to act in the same way. In healthcare ethics, this means that duties and rights are taken into account in our ethical decision-making.

Kant's deontological approach to ethics

Kant's main discussion of ethics can be found in *Groundwork for the Metaphysics of Morals* (1997), *The Critique of Practical Reason* (1909) and *The Metaphysics of Morals* ((1991). The first of these is generally taken to encapsulate Kant's novel contribution to the discussion of ethics. Throughout his work on ethics, Kant takes a contrary view to those who claim that we can determine what is morally good by an appeal to the good, which he claims we cannot know, as well as those – such as virtue ethicists – who claim that the end of ethical behaviour is happiness. The latter, he thinks, cannot adequately be established. Kant provides us with a view of ethics that he believes is based on reason, the distinguishing mark of a human being. He distrusts emotion, holding that doing what is good is an imperative of reason: the recognition of doing what is right and the will to do this, irrespective of how one feels about what one has to do. While utilitarianism conceives of morality in terms of the interests of those with a stake in what one is proposing to do, and in terms of whether good is maximised, the Kantian argues that moral standards exist independently of utilitarian ends. An act or rule is right, the deontologist maintains, if it satisfies the demands of an overriding non-utilitarian principle or principles of obligation. That is, actions are right or wrong not because of their consequences, but because one has a duty or obligation to others to act in that way. Thus keeping a promise, being loyal to one's friends, repaying a debt and so on are duties or obligations, which it is right that one should carry out. For this reason, Kant's approach to ethics is termed deontological.

For the healthcare practitioner, there is something appealing in Kant's approach, as it proposes that moral questions concerning the treatment of patients can be determined by an appeal to reason, rather than to intuitions about what is the right thing to do or a process of weighing up everyone's interests. It appears to give us an objective answer to our questions about whether we should override a patient's preference for a particular treatment when it is clear that it is not in his interest. It proposes that our decisions about what actions to take can be determined through an appeal to rational principles of obligation that are applicable in every situation. If it is our obligation to treat patients, then whatever our preferences or theirs may be, it is the right thing to do.

Central to Kant's conception of ethics is his conviction that ethics – like everything else in the world – is governed by laws and that these laws are based on metaphysics, by which he means that they are grounded in *a priori* principles or judgements. That is, knowing what we ought to do is not only a matter of experience, but of acting according to previously established principles that can be known through reason (Korsgaard, 1996). In *Groundwork for the Metaphysics of Morals*, Kant (1997) says that his aim is nothing more than the search for and establishment of the supreme principle of morality. In addition, he also seeks to justify the use of this principle by human beings, and to apply it in practical situations. From a practical viewpoint, it is not enough that we establish such a principle, as Kant well recognises, since it also needs to be able to be applied in the many different situations that we face in the world. Kant (1991) works out the details of application in *The Metaphysics of Morals*, elaborating the ideas he sets out in the *Groundwork*. In Kant's system, the 'free choice' of the rational agent becomes a hallmark of ethical decision-making. What Kant connects are things that must be present for someone to be a moral agent: first, the capacity to comply with the requirements of a moral law, and second, the capacity to be capable of impulses that could induce them not to comply[1] – that is, an agent capable of free choice. Moral decisions have to be considered not just in the light of the supreme principle of morality, but also in relation to an understanding of duties that we owe to others, and those that arise as a result of the requirements of moral virtue. Furthermore, we have to be capable of making a choice.

Kant says that everyone has to accept that if a law is to hold morally – that is, as the reason for an obligation that we must meet – it has to hold absolutely. For example, the rule or law 'don't lie' holds not just for human beings, but for all other rational beings. This will be the case for other moral laws. This means, he continues, that the reason for the obligation is not dependent on the nature of human beings or the particular situation, but is grounded *a priori* – that is, prior to and independent of experience – in concepts of pure reason. He acknowledges that there may be other rules based on our experience that we might universalise, but these can never be moral laws – only practical rules. Moral rules or laws differ from other principles that depend on experience in some way, and moral philosophy is based entirely on concepts in pure reason. He notes, however, that the application of such laws will still require judgement sharpened by experience, because we need to be able to know cases in which particular laws apply and those in which they do not. Moreover, experience also provides us with an understanding of the will, and how we can fulfil moral laws, since human beings – although capable of the idea of practical pure reason – are affected by so many inclinations that they find it difficult to apply them in concrete situations (Kant, 1997).

Hypothetical and categorical imperatives

Kant (1997) believes that everything in nature works according to laws, and only a rational being with a will is capable of acting in accordance with such laws. The will itself is nothing but practical reason, since we need to use reason in deciding what to do. This will be the case whatever it is that we want to do, as whatever we desire to obtain will require us to act in order to get it, and that means working out how to get it. It is possible, Kant admits, that the will is swayed by various inclinations, and so is not in conformity with objective reason. This means that, though reason can tell us what actions are in conformity with moral laws, a will that is swayed by desires will not necessarily act according to them. Will acting in accordance with a rational moral principle, however, is necessarily acting according to a command of reason, and the formula of a command is called an imperative. Standardly, an imperative is expressed by an 'ought' (Kant, 1997).

The central question for Kant is, 'What ought I to do?' He distinguishes between hypothetical imperatives – such as, 'If I want to be a great musician then I ought to practise playing my instrument', 'If I want to be a competent nurse then I ought to study hard', 'If I want to lose weight, I will need to go on a diet', and what he calls the categorical imperative. Hypothetical imperatives tell us what we ought to do, provided that we have the relevant desire or want. Categorical imperatives, on the other hand, are binding on rational agents simply because they are rational in their orientation. Hypothetical imperatives simply enjoin us to do what is necessary if we want to achieve a particular goal. For example, if we want to have enough money to buy a house, then we ought to save the deposit. The action of saving is only necessary if we want to buy a house; if we change our minds, then we are not obliged to continue saving (Kant, 1997). Categorical imperatives, on the other hand, oblige us to act, since they represent actions that are objectively necessary if we are to conform to what is objectively good. For example, 'If it is my duty to give this patient this medication to save his life, then I ought to give it to him' and, 'If it is my duty to give my customers the right change, then I ought to give it to them'. In these examples, the strength of the 'ought' is much greater, since an obligation to conform to a moral principle in the presence of a good will compels us to act in accordance with it. To act otherwise is to do evil, which results in harm to another or to self.

The good will

Kant constructs the principles of ethics according to the dictates of reason, identifying a good will as the only unconditional good. The good will is the extra ingredient that enables us to act morally. From the outset, Kant proposes that the metaphysics of morals has to examine the idea and the principles of a possible pure will. He is interested only in the idea of a pure will, and how this would work in relation to morality. He is not interested in the acts and conditions of human willing, which are about the psychology of willing, but about what is required for a good moral action. It is the good will that is the only thing that can be called good in the world without qualification. One reason for this is that an act cannot be called morally good unless it is done for the sake of the moral law, not merely in conformity with the law. It is acting in accordance with the good will that makes it good (Kant, 1997).

Kant believes that a good will is the only unconditional good because anything else that we might consider good can be used for evil. Thus wealth, and mental and physical health, can be used immorally. We can, for example, use wealth to gain power over others, to coerce them, and we can certainly abuse our mental and physical health. Hence knowing what is good – even what the basic human goods are – does not mean that we will do what is right. There are many talents, such as intelligence, wit and judgement, as well as qualities of temperament, he says, that we might possess, but unless the will that is to make use of them is good, they can become bad because of the way we use (or abuse) them. The same, he notes, is true of power, riches, honour and even health. Possession of these can lead to arrogance and pride, unless our actions are moderated by a good will that corrects the tendencies to evil. Kant (1997) proposes that possession of a good will is a prerequisite to being worthy of happiness.

Kant observes that we do not always succeed in carrying out what we want to achieve, despite our best intentions and efforts, so we cannot be morally condemned just for failing. On the other hand, we cannot expect to be praised for unintentionally doing something good. Intentions or a good will formed with the desire to do what one ought to do – that is, to be motivated by a sense of duty to do what is right – are what constitutes the intrinsically good. If I am motivated to do what is right, and having determined what that is, then a good will ensures that I will do what is right. What is important for Kant is discovering what principles can be adopted by a plurality of agents without specifying anything particular about an agent's desires or their social relations. The main consideration is in determining what is right to do. This is not a simple matter of doing what we think is right, or what interests us at a particular time, but doing what our duty or our obligation to do happens to be. Morality, for Kant, begins with the rejection of non-universalisability and the adoption of the categorical imperative. The three formulations of the categorical imperative are not equivalent to each other, but elaborate Kant's conception of morality as being universal (Korsgaard, 1996).

Duty and the categorical imperative

For Kant, duty connects with the categorical imperative in the case of moral actions. We have already mentioned some examples of duties, but these in themselves do not define what is meant by a duty. If it is our duty to give patients their medication or treatment, this is because we are healthcare professionals, and overseeing the medication and treatment of patients is part of our professional role. There is nothing in this that is especially a moral action, though neglect of our duties could be a moral matter, as our patients could become seriously ill as a result of our negligence. Professional duties, conduct statements, codes of ethics or position descriptions present a type of duty framework for the health professional, but Kant thinks about duties more broadly. He says, for example, that to be beneficent is a duty and to assure one's own happiness is a duty (Kant, 1997). Here Kant compares someone who is kind-hearted, and so acts generously, with someone who is largely indifferent to the sufferings of others, but nevertheless acts generously. He thinks that it is the second case that is more meritorious, since the person acts from duty and not from inclination. We might want to disagree with Kant about this, but his point is that sometimes acting in a morally good way can be very demanding, and we should regard someone who does the right thing when it is difficult as more praiseworthy than someone who does what is good without much effort.

Kant (1997: 12–13) defines duty as follows:

- He points to the command in scripture to love one's neighbour, and even one's enemy, as an example of duty. Here, he says, love as an inclination cannot be commanded, but is a beneficence that comes from doing one's duty. It is a practical love, not a pathological one, because it lies in the good will and not in inclinations or feelings. Because this kind of love is actioned by the will, it can be commanded, whereas love that arises from inclinations and feelings cannot. That is, love that arises from passion is not rational, not under the control of the will, and we act on impulses. Duty is therefore a type of practical love that we express for other human beings, which is not connected to any feelings we might have for them.
- Second, an action from duty will have moral worth not because of the purposes to be attained by the action, but because of the moral principle according to which the decision to act was taken. This is important, since duty has nothing to do with the consequences of the action, but rather with a moral principle that commands our adherence if we want to act morally.
- Third, and as a consequence of the first two conditions, a duty is a necessity that results from respect for the moral law. That is, if a duty is practical love of neighbour and adherence to a moral principle, it follows that, in order to respect the moral law, we are obliged to act according to what duty demands of us.

Kant (1997: 14) says that if we act from duty, we eliminate the influence of our inclinations and feelings, as well as any other thing that can distract our will from the moral law and the pure respect that we should have for this practical law, even if it goes against all our inclinations. What this entails is that we should only act according to a rule, principle or maxim that we would also want to become a universal law binding on everyone. What Kant calls a maxim is the subjective principle of our willing. That is, it is the rule we follow when we will or determine to do something; it is what moves us to act. In moral action, however, we cannot simply follow a rule of our own, since Kant says that morality has to be universal – so the same for everyone. The rule or principle we follow has to be universal and objective. All rational beings, if they follow the dictates of reason, will have the same objective principle or moral rule to guide their decision-making. Of course, Kant realises that human beings may let their desires influence them in their moral decision-making, so he is at pains to argue that the universal principle guiding moral decision-making has to be both objective and universal, as well as the result of rational reasoning. Hence he says that the objective principle that serves subjectively as the practical principle for all rational beings if reason had complete control over the faculty of desire is the practical law, and is a maxim in a special way.

Kant provides us with an example of what he means by acting from duty. There is a difference between acting from self-interest and acting out of duty. A shopkeeper may give an inexperienced customer or a child the correct change because he believes it is his duty to act honestly, or because he is feeling kindly towards the inexperienced customer or likes children, or because he thinks that if he doesn't his reputation will suffer and he will lose customers. Kant says that only the first of these is a moral action, since the shopkeeper acts out of duty. Similarly, if a nurse changes her patient's dressings because she believes it is her duty to ensure that they are replaced by clean ones, or she feels sorry for her patient or, if she doesn't, she could lose her job. Again, only the first can be considered a moral action. The meaning of the first formulation of the categorical imperative is now clear, since it specifies not only the universal nature of the moral principles in accord with which we should act, but also its binding nature. If acting in a particular way is objectively and rationally our duty, then it follows that we are bound to act in accord with the objective moral rule that directs us to act in a particular way. If it is a universal rule that our duty is to look after our patients, then if we consider the situation objectively and rationally, according to the good will, we will change their dressings when they need to be changed.

The first formulation of the categorical imperative

The first formulation of the categorical imperative thus arises out of Kant's understanding of how duty ought to compel us to act according to what is required by a good will and by adherence to moral law. Kant (1997: 15) says, 'I ought never to act except in such a way that I could also will that my maxim should become a universal law.' The maxim or first formulation of the categorical imperative can be illustrated by an example. Suppose we hold that we should always keep our promises. For this to be a universal moral rule, we would expect everyone to keep their promises. There are difficulties with such a moral rule as, plausibly, if we promise to repay $50 we have borrowed, then the expectation is that if our rule is to keep our promises then we would repay the $50 as promised. Moreover, if we loaned $50 to someone, we would expect that they would keep their promise to repay the loan. Let us suppose now that we take an opposite view. Suppose we want 'never keep your promises' to be a universal law accepted by everyone. This means that though we can simply ignore requests to repay the borrowed $50, we cannot expect anyone else to repay any money they borrowed from us either. If no promises are ever to be kept, then the concept of a promise becomes empty, since no one ever keeps them. The resulting social chaos would be devastating, and it is easy to see that such a universal law would destroy itself.[2]

There is, however, a difficulty with the first formulation of the categorical imperative. The problem is that it is too wide and too unqualified (Pojman, 2005). Suppose, for example, that we hold the following rule: 'Nurses should always wear a recognisable pink uniform.' This rule is universalisable without contradiction. Remembering that this is a rule that we would will that everyone – including ourselves – would be required to obey as a universal maxim, it clearly would fit the first formulation. We are happy to require others to wear pink uniforms, and prepared to wear them ourselves. This is, however, a trivial law, and arguably is not a moral law, so should not be considered a serious objection to the first formulation of the categorical imperative. A more serious objection is raised if the content is moral, however. Suppose I hold the following rule: 'Use pornography for sexual pleasure.' The rule is universalisable, since we will that everyone – including ourselves – would be required to obey this rule as a universal maxim. No contradiction arises, nor is the rule trivial.

Unlike the rule about promising, the rule does not lead to any self-contradiction in its application. Whether it would lead to bad consequences is another matter, but since Kant's theory is non-consequential,[3] we cannot plausibly appeal to consequences in the same way as the consequentialist can. We have to show why the rule is a bad one using Kant's understanding of what makes a rule a moral principle. There are other examples that we could find of a similar kind.

Another difficulty is the requirement of the first formulation to be exceptionalness. It is to hold for all people. For example, if we hold the moral principle, 'Don't lie', this holds for all people and in all situations, since it is a universal maxim. Suppose, however, that a woman rings your doorbell and asks for your help, as her violently jealous boyfriend is chasing her with a view to killing her for an imagined indiscretion. You agree, and hide her in your attic. Moments later, the violent boyfriend, axe in hand, rings your doorbell and asks you whether his girlfriend is in your house. Kant says you should tell the truth, 'Yes, she is in the house.' Intuitively, apart from concerns about opening your door to someone wielding an axe, this does not seem morally right. One reason for this is that it contravenes another moral principle, 'Protect innocent human life'. If both are taken to be exceptionalness, there does not seem to be any simple way under Kant's formulation to decide what to do.

The second formulation of the categorical imperative

Kant is aware of the difficulties and moves to a second formulation of the categorical imperative. He arrives at the second formulation by reflecting on the kind of being that would place itself under the requirements of the first formulation of the categorical imperative. He proposes that it is a rational being, since it is only such a being whose will is capable of acting in conformity with moral laws. Rational beings, he asserts, have absolute worth, and are ends in themselves, so are fitting grounds for determinate laws (Kant, 1997). That is, rational beings are the justification for determinate laws. All human beings, he contends, exist as an end in themselves, never as a means to be used by another's will for their own purposes. Kant distinguishes human beings from animals – that is, beings that exist in nature, but have no rational nature – arguing that while these have a relative worth, human beings – because they are rational beings and so are persons – are ends in themselves, and so may not be used merely as means. Rational nature exists as an end in itself, and this applies to all human beings. The second formulation of the categorical imperative given by Kant (1997: 37–8) is: 'So act that you use humanity, whether in your own person or in the person of any other, always at the same time as an end and never merely as a means.' This formulation of the categorical imperative has had the greatest impact, since it demands that we treat humanity in our own persons or in the person of any other never simply as a means, but always at the same time as an end. This is a highly articulated version of a demand for respect for persons. According to this formulation, we do not demand that everyone adopt the same maxims, but ask that when we act, we do so in such a way that others are not prevented from being free to choose how to act for themselves. Kant says that we cannot use another as a thing or a tool for our own ends, nor can we act in such a way that it is impossible for another to act.

The second formulation obliges us to support one another's capacities to act, to adopt maxims and to pursue our particular ends. This means that we cannot refuse to develop our own capacities either, since to do so constitutes a failure to respect oneself as well as humanity in general, which we are also obliged to support because to do otherwise means that we are impeding the pursuit of others of their ends. Kant does not think that we can be indifferent to others, even though we could formulate a universal principle according to which we could will others to treat us in the same way – namely, with indifference.

The categorical imperative, in its second formulation, explicitly recognises that human beings are not only rational beings, but also physical beings with emotions, and that this adds a special dimension to human morality. Kant's understanding of persons, however, is impersonal, recognising only that they are ends against which we should not act, and his view of morality is often taken to be an ethics for relations between strangers (Sullivan, 1994). Kant, however, did not see that all that was required was that we should merely avoid others and be indifferent to them; he required us to have positive duties to others as well. The claim that persons are 'ends in themselves' means that they should be regarded as having intrinsic worth – an idea Kant adopts from Christianity. Kant, however, wants to construct a moral view based on reason, not faith, so needs some other way of understanding this notion.

Although it is true that, as dependent beings, we have to rely on others and their skills and abilities, it does not mean that we can treat them as means only. When we rely on a mechanic to fix our car, we treat them as a means; however, this is not wrong, since the mechanic's worth is not determined by their usefulness to us. The individual person has an absolute and irreplaceable dignity, and so cannot be treated as only a means or merely a source of satisfaction of our desires. We are obliged to respect the person because they are a person, irrespective of whether they carried out something that we wanted them to do. We respect individuals irrespective of whether they are morally good or bad, for respect is owed because they are autonomous beings with the capacity to develop a morally good will.

What is also stressed in the second formulation is that we need to be moral because this is required of us in order to live up to the dignity we have as persons. Furthermore, whenever we act immorally, we treat ourselves as mere things, and so do not give ourselves respect. Kant condemned suicide because it meant that we would have under-valued our self-worth and had failed to fulfil the positive duty to perfect ourselves. Kant believes that we have other negative duties to ourselves too. Respect for ourselves means that we do not indulge in over-eating, for example, nor use drugs, since our abilities to think and act rationally and morally are impaired.

Just as we have the right to the respect of others, so too they have the right to respect from us. Kant's second formulation recognises this, but Kant wants to move further than just a recognition of negative duties to others – that is, refraining from harming them, or interfering with what they might want to do. He says that we also have a positive obligation to recognise and promote, as far as we are able, the happiness of others. This does not mean that we are responsible for another's happiness or moral character, but it means that in our pursuit of happiness, we contribute where we can to the moral happiness of others. Kant summarised this obligation as a 'law of love'. This is, however, moral love, which is not an emotion, but rather a practical attitude to how we should act towards others. Our moral obligation to contribute to the happiness of others rests fundamentally on respect for them as persons, rather than on their happiness being of special concern to us.

Universal benevolence or well-wishing requires only that we wish others well. Beneficence, on the other hand, requires us to actively help others. Kant recognises the limits of this, for we do not violate the maxim of concern for others by choosing to help some persons rather than others. Because human beings are limited in their resources, this requirement means that we cannot contribute to the well-being of everyone – only God can do that.

It is evident that this reformulation adds something substantive to the first purely formal formulation of the categorical imperative. Kant (1991) viewed the second formulation as a restatement of the first, but it is easy to see that it adds some further content. We are to treat ourselves, as well as others, with respect. This would rule out the rule, 'Use pornography for sexual pleasure' as a universal moral rule to follow, since pornography degrades human beings, and uses them as merely a means to the end of sexual gratification. It also rules out using human beings as merely a means to an end. It does not end our difficulties entirely, since obviously – as the example of the mechanic shows – we regularly use human beings as means to ends in our daily lives. Some further instances are provided by the following. For example, the surgeon who operates on us is a means to the end of restoration to health. Although Kant would agree that the surgeon is a means, he would argue that they are not merely a means, but an intrinsic end as well. The problem is it is not entirely clear how to draw the distinction between treating someone as merely a means or as a means in a legitimate context. We visit the nutritionist to help us plan our weight-loss regimen, so they are a means to the end we have in mind – namely, weight loss. It seems we could also say legitimately that the nutritionist is merely the means of getting the right meals planned; the rest of the diet is up to us to implement. Kant has in mind something more: that we treat the dietician with respect because they are a human being with intrinsic worth and because they are a rational being.

This, however, will still not be enough, since there are serious cases where it is unclear what treating others as ends in themselves amounts to. For example, suppose you are an intensive care nurse and you are caring for a seriously ill patient, who pleads with you to give him more morphine because he is in pain. You are aware that he had received his last dose only an hour previously, and that the anaesthesiologist had visited the patient and calcu-lated the various doses of different drugs for pain relief. Allowing the patient to suffer until the next dose of morphine is due does not seem to be treating him as an end in himself, since you leave him to his suffering. On the other hand, seeking out the anaesthesiologist to provide the go-ahead for an extra dose might also not be in the patient's interest. If, later, the patient requests to end his life because of the unendurable pain he is suffering, you are then faced with a challenge regarding the application of the second formulation. This is because someone who is suffering greatly, is incontinent and is unable to do something for himself can be seen as lacking dignity proper to a human being, so if he, as an autonomous human being, determines that his life should end, then respect for persons could be taken to mean that we should assist him to realise his final wish.

Kant, however, does not agree with this understanding of the application of the second formulation since, in his view, a human being has absolute intrinsic worth. He begins by proposing that someone who has suicide on his mind has to ask himself whether his proposed action can be consistent with the idea of humanity as an end in itself. His response is that the proposed action cannot be consistent with it since, in trying to escape the situation of suffering, the individual makes use of a person (himself) as merely a means to maintain a tolerable situation up to the end of life. In all our actions, we must not use either ourselves or another as merely a means to an end. This is because human beings are not things, but must in all their actions be regarded as ends in themselves (Kant, 1997). Kant rejects the idea that we can depart life at our discretion and time of choosing, because in this very courage of not fearing death, we should be aware of something that we should value more highly than our own life: the absolute worth of being a being capable of such powerful authority in decision-making, and so knowing that it is wrong to deprive ourselves of life. Life cannot be renounced as long as we live, for we are always subject to duties – not only to ourselves, but also to others. Starkly, Kant says that to annihilate the subject of morality in our own person is to destroy the existence of morality in the world, as far as one can (Kant, 1991) What confers value on the judgement that life should be tolerable is the being whose destruction is being proposed; hence the destruction of the reason for morality is being destroyed. For Kant, our obligations run very deep, and our absolute worth lies in being ends in ourselves, which includes being the bearers and preservers of morality itself – in short, of our rational nature or humanity. Our last duty is to uphold the existence of morality in the world.

The third formulation of the categorical imperative

This leads to a consideration of Kant's third formulation of the categorical imperative. Kant notes that human beings are ends in themselves, and that the natural end of human beings is happiness. We have already noted that we have duties – not only to ourselves, but also to others – and Kant wonders whether we have any obligation to contribute to the happiness of others. His response is to propose that inherent to being ends in ourselves is the recognition that others are not only ends in themselves but that, in contributing to their happiness, we contribute to their fulfilment as ends – that is, to their humanity. At the same time, we also contribute to our humanity, and so to our own happiness. What Kant means by humanity in this context is not entirely clear, but one interpretation is that Kant means our rational nature, our capacity to take a rational interest in something, to decide, under the influence of reason, that something is desirable and worthy of pursuit or realisation, that it is to be deemed important or valuable as an end for its own sake (Korsgaard, 1996). This rational nature – humanity – has absolute worth, and so is the ground of a practical law (Kant, 1997).

Recognition that others are also rational beings – ends in themselves with the same rational nature or humanity as we have – leads Kant to propose what he calls the kingdom of ends. Given that all rational beings stand under the law that a person is to treat their own self and all others never as merely a means but always at the same time as an end in themselves, they will, once we have abstracted their personal ends, have in common objective laws – that is, a kingdom of ends (Kant, 1997). This amounts to recognition that each individual person is a rational being who can autonomously decide on their own actions. At the same time, Kant recognises that we also have to contribute to the development of our humanity, and this is a common endeavour. We require the support of each other to be able to do this.

The third formula presents us with a moral vision of our final and comprehensive collective destiny, thereby satisfying our rational need for an ultimate goal. It is Kant's response to the question of what it is that a person can hope for if they act in a moral manner. Kant says that acting morally entails not just a duty to be concerned with one's own moral good, but the good of all, and this means that one has to strive to realise a collective good, which is not just an aggregation of the good of individuals. What Kant seems to have in mind is something like the establishment of the Kingdom of God, though Kant refers to this third form of moral ideal as the 'kingdom of ends'; however, this is not quite what Kant had in mind.

Kant's moral community – the 'kingdom of ends' – cannot be regarded as being itself the ultimate good except in a certain sense. The ultimate good for Kant is the good will as the expression of a rational nature. Human beings possess a rational nature – humanity – but this is far from perfect, and it is the role of each human being to develop this nature. This is to be done in the company of others also endowed with a rational nature. Since the good will is itself good, its development will also lead to other kinds of good, including the ability to love and respect others. Ultimately, human beings serve the good by doing their duty rather than striving for happiness. What Kant means by this is that happiness begins in first recognising our duties to others.

Conclusion

Kant regards the three formulations as statements of the very same law, but showing at the same time a progression in how it is to be understood. The first formulation expresses the universality of the maxim; the second deals with the plurality of those covered by it; and the third presents the totality of the system of ends – that is, the moral community. A strong theme in Kant's thought is the importance of reason in helping us determine how to act. That is, a rational being will act in accord with the categorical imperative, since to do otherwise would be contradictory, as well as wrong. It fails, in addition, to treat others as not merely means, but rather ends in themselves, because it prioritises individual goals ahead of duties owed to others. Moreover, a law that is contradictory cannot be shared by a plurality of rational beings, and so cannot lead to the realisation of the kingdom of ends.

Although criticisms can be made of Kant's moral theory – for example, that it is too rigid because it insists on the absoluteness of moral rules, that it finds no place for the emotions, that rules which are universal are likely to be too general to work in specific situations and conflicts between absolutes are difficult to handle – it centres moral action, and so responsibility, clearly on individual actors. The great virtue of Kant's formulation of ethics is that he proposes that ethics can be founded on reason. Acting morally not only involves doing what is right, but what is right can be determined by reflecting on what it would be rational to do for any other rational agent in similar circumstances. A universal ethics also implies the recognition that there are other rational agents, and that in giving reasons for acting, these must satisfy universal principles.

Reflective exercises

9.1 What kind of healthcare practitioner would you prefer to treat you – one who is empathetic, but not particularly good at doing their job, or one who always conscientiously does their duty well, but has little empathy? Discuss.

9.2 This chapter presents the following statement, 'There is a difference between acting from self-interest and acting out of duty.' Provide an example from your clinical practice where self-interest and duty may conflict, and result in an ethical dilemma. What moral and professional frameworks might guide you in moral reasoning in this scenario?

9.3 What is a duty? Suppose the government legislates that euthanasia is to be legalised and that all medical practitioners are required to comply with any reasonable request to assist someone to die. Is there a duty to comply with the law? Discuss.

9.4 Why should we treat rational autonomous human beings as having absolute worth? What implications does this Kantian notion have for persons who may not be able to be rational, such as those experiencing altered consciousness, mental illness or advanced cognitive decline such as dementia?

9.5 What are the main distinctions between the three formulations of Kant's categorical imperative? Summarise each of the formulations and provide a clinical example for each.

9.6 The second formulation of the categorical imperative given by Kant is, 'So act that you use humanity, whether in your own person or in the person of any other, always at the same time as an end and never merely as a means.' What, then, may be a Kantian perspective on the moral rightness or wrongness of a couple entering into a contract for a surrogate child?

9.7 Suppose a patient objects to a blood transfusion on moral grounds, even though we know it will save his life. Do we have a duty, as a healthcare practitioner, to give him a transfusion? What would Kant argue is the morally right thing to do given this scenario?

9.8 Kant's second formation of the categorical imperative states that whenever we act immorally we treat ourselves as mere things, and so do not give ourselves respect. What, then, would be Kant's reasoning of a health professional assisting a patient to end their life through providing the means to suicide? Would Kantian reasoning change when the action of assisted suicide and the health professional's involvement is legalised? Reflect on this second formation statement with relation to assisted suicide and the collective implications for health professional groups that willingly engage in assisted suicide practice. Do you think there could be a public loss of respect for certain health professional groups that engage in such actions?

Notes

1. The first condition is obvious enough: someone who is not a moral agent cannot be subject to the moral law. The second criterion is a criterion of freedom. Only those who are capable of actual choice can be considered to have freedom of choice (Gregor, 1991: 4).

2. It should be stressed that this is because the universal rule is self-contradictory, as the concept of promising becomes empty not because of the consequences – even though it is obvious that they would be serious if the concept of promising became unusable.

3. Some would argue that Kant's moral theory is similar in some ways to rule utilitarianism. See, for example, Tännsjö (2002: 59). Hare (1997: 147ff.) also tentatively supposes that utilitarians and Kant are not as far apart as is often thought.

References

Gregor, M. (1991). Introduction. In I. Kant, *The metaphysics of morals*. Cambridge: Cambridge University Press.

Hare, R. M. (1997). *Sorting out ethics*. Oxford: Clarendon Press.

Kant, I. (1909). *The critique of practical reason and other works on the theory of ethics*. Tr. Thomas Kingsmill Abbott. London: Longmans, Green and Co.

—— (1991). *The metaphysics of morals*, intro., trans. and notes M. Gregor. Cambridge: Cambridge University Press.

—— (1997). *Groundwork for the metaphysics of morals*, trans. and ed. M. Gregor. Cambridge: Cambridge University Press.

Korsgaard, C. M. (1996). *Creating the kingdom of ends*. Cambridge: Cambridge University Press.

Pojman, L. P. (2005). *How should we live?* Belmont, CA: Wadsworth/ Thomson Learning.

Sullivan, R. J. (1994). *An introduction to Kant's ethics*. Cambridge: Cambridge University Press.

Tännsjö, T. (2002). *Understanding ethics: An introduction to moral theory*. Edinburgh: Edinburgh University Press.

10 A historical analysis of feminism and an application to contemporary healthcare ethics

Joanne Grainger

In her book *Feminist Politics and Human Nature*, Alison Jaggar (1983) argues that, in some form or another, feminism has always existed. For as long as women have experienced social, political or cultural subordination, there have been either individual or communal women who have resisted this reduction in status. Over the last two centuries, a visible and organised feminist movement has emerged. This chapter will present a historical timeline of feminist theory that will include an identification of several proto-feminists, and explore the social, cultural and ethical foundations of contemporary feminist theory. The three main 'waves' of feminism will be analysed, key writers and activists in these areas identified, and some workable definitions of relevant broad terms presented. Emancipation, suffragettes, radical feminism, liberation movement, care ethics and global feminism are fundamental terms that will be explored in this chapter. It will be argued that contemporary feminist theory is predominately a Western construct and that for application in non-Western, indigenous and culturally and linguistically diverse cultures, theoretical adaptation should be considered.

In the final section of the chapter, an application of one element of contemporary feminist theory will be presented in connection with healthcare
ethics: relational autonomy. A case study involving the care of a woman with
an unplanned pregnancy will be highlighted to assist with the application of
relational autonomy and the connection with healthcare ethical reasoning.

A historical review of the origins of contemporary feminism

The claim of natural sexual distinction as being the foundation for women's
inferior status in society was initially challenged during the eighteenth century.
Anglo-Irish writer Mary Wollstonecraft (1995) is recognised as one of the
'mothers' of contemporary feminism. She reacted against the likes of the
French writer Rousseau and other English writers, who saw women as being
restricted to primarily a role within the private sphere. Her best known work
is *A Vindication of the Rights of Women*, originally published in 1792. This
treatise was distributed in the Enlightenment period of English and Western
history during the height of the Industrial Revolution, when other reform
movements – such as that for the abolition of slavery – were prominent.

Changes to the traditional economic status of the family were significant
in this period. In the United Kingdom, feudalism had been replaced by the
centralised nation-state, resulting in a decline in the economic and political
significance of the family (Jaggar, 1983). New post-industrial democratic ideas
of autonomy and equality challenged traditional societal assumptions of
women being subordinate to men. In this era of dramatic social change,
Wollstonecraft argued women deserved the same fundamental rights as men.
Her primary focus of equality related to access to education for women that
enabled them to develop independence of mind and become active contributors
to the progress of society (Bowden & Mummery, 2009).

From exploring the universal rights of humanity to outlining the particular
rights of women, Wollstonecraft (1995) affirmed the need for women to be
self-determining and accountable, and to develop an individual sense of worth
through education, and social and civic engagement. Through combining a
natural rights argument with justice, Wollstonecraft demanded that women
share civic and political rights with men, but also that these rights must be
applied to relations within the family. For Wollstonecraft, women were autonomous and rational agents, and emancipation from social subordination was

possible through traditional institutional opportunities such as education, employment and engagement in civil and political rights.

Despite living nearly a century apart, nineteenth-century English philosopher John Stuart Mill's libertarian views are analogous with many of those presented by Wollstonecraft. Coole (1988: 133) affirms Mill as 'the most significant liberal thinker' in history by presenting a political and social theory for the emancipation of women. In his work *The Subjection of Women* (1869), Mill argued that there was a need to put laws into place to ensure the legal protection of women and social empowerment. For Mill, advocacy of sexual equality was a key feature of his political and economic pursuit of a more liberal society. Mill (1869: 56) stated:

> It may be asserted without scruple, that no other class of dependants have had their character so entirely distorted from its natural proportions by their relation with their masters [than women].

Through his social and political advocacy of and for women, Mill aimed to measure and review differences between the sexes in order to better argue for equal legal and social justice for women in traditional social institutions. In *The Subjection of Women*, Mill appealed to men's humanity to reaffirm the inherent dignity of a woman, and argued for political and social equality in nineteenth-century England. Like Wollstonecraft, Mill could be viewed as a proto-feminist, as he helped to lay down the political, legal and social foundations for the first wave of feminism that would become active a century or so later.

The three 'waves' of contemporary feminism

The journey of twenty-first-century feminism had its origins in Europe and the United States in the late nineteenth century. Feminist academic Karen Offen (1988) argues that it is essential to review the historical foundations of modern feminist political and social theory in order to re-examine and present a new conceptualisation of the term. Such conceptual and historical analysis can also provide academic scholars with foundations for responding to contemporary social, cultural and political issues that concern women, and also other vulnerable and disempowered members of our community. Therefore, continuing this historical exploration of feminist theoretical origins, the different 'waves' of feminist theory will be analysed. The metaphor of 'waves' has essentially become a trope for understanding and describing what seem to be the distinct periods of contemporary feminist thought (Howie & Tauchert, 2007). Despite this figurative categorisation of these periods as 'waves', each distinct divisions is useful for undertaking a broad introductory historical analysis of feminism.

The first wave of feminism arose from the context of social change fostered by industrialisation and liberalism, and was set predominantly in the late nineteenth and early twentieth centuries. The primary concern for feminists in this era were to proclaim equal opportunity for women in society (Krolokke & Scott-Sorensen, 2012). The early liberal and human rights foundations of feminism laid down by Wollstonecraft and Mill were used as a scaffold for the rise of the suffragette movement. The term 'suffragette' was originally coined by a British newspaper as a derogatory term depicting militant activists. Suffragettes were predominately white, middle-class, well-educated women who organised meetings and public demonstrations to voice their primary argument: that women and men were equal in legal terms, and therefore to deny women the ability to vote was essentially to deny women full citizenship status. First-wave feminists Emmeline Pankhurst, Sylvia Pankhurst and Emily Wilding Davidson were part of a group of British women who pressed for social reform and the right for women to vote. In Australia, the suffragette movement pressed for women's right to vote at the same time as their British sisters were agitating for reform. Australia was the first country in the world to give women both the right to vote in federal elections and the right to be elected to parliament. Key Australian suffragette instigators included Vida Goldstein, Edith Cowan, Rose Scott and Mary Lee (Vanstone, 2002). Interestingly, it was in New Zealand in 1893 that the first women in a Western democracy were able to vote. After several decades of suffragette campaigning, British women over the age of 30 were finally granted this right in 1918.

In the time between the first- and second-'wave' periods, several key historical developments influenced the feminist movement's upward social and political trajectory. From the late 1930s to the mid-1940s, women entered the workforce in record numbers in Western countries that were at war. 'Womanpower' became integral to the rapidly expanding defence industries, as more men left this form of employment for active military service. Women therefore assumed jobs and roles that had previously been considered men's work. A key marketing figure promoting the role of women in defence industries during this time was 'Rosie the Riveter' (Gluck, 1988). Despite most women returning to domestic duties after the war (whether they wanted to or not), an increased respect for women's work capacities and capabilities was established. Indeed, 'Rosie the Riveter' became the iconic image of the radical feminist and female same sex movement prominent in the second wave of feminism (Gluck, 1988). Another key historical moment was the publication of *The Second Sex* by French existentialist philosopher Simone de Beauvoir, which has been viewed as a feminist manifesto. First published in English in 1952, this 700-plus page composition on male theorisation of 'woman' and the challenges of women's lived experience in contemporary Western society launched de Beauvoir's reputation as a feminist. De Beauvoir's primary thesis in *The Second Sex* was that men fundamentally oppress women by characterising them, on every level, as the 'Other' – or the second and subordinate sex to men. For de Beauvoir, by defining woman exclusively as the 'Other' sex, her humanity and dignity are denied. De Beauvoir provides insight into the economic underpinnings of female subordination, and argued that for women to be truly liberated and self-determining, a woman must work to support herself. In her text, de Beauvoir discusses how contraception and legal access to abortion can free women from the 'tyranny' of pregnancy and domestic life. From the late 1950s and early 1960s, de Beauvoir's *The Second Sex* (1952) became a guide for the theoretical yet practical 'birth' of the second-wave feminist movement.

The second wave of feminism can be separated into two distinct periods, with the first period being from late 1960s to the mid-1970s, and the second being the 1980s. Radical feminism and the women's liberation movement are key features of this earlier period, with relationships between men and women deeply politicised. Feminist texts such as Germaine Greer's (1970) *The Female Eunuch*, Juliet Mitchell's (1974) *Psychoanalysis and Feminism*, Betty Friedan's (1964) *The Feminine Mystique* and Kate Millett's (1969) *Sexual Politics* primarily argued that a woman's sexuality is disconnected from the social obligations of marriage and motherhood. Strongly aligned with Liberalism and socialist Marxism, the demands for equal pay at work, a breakdown in gender division in access to education and the ability of women to choose whatever work that they desired were key areas of focus for these radical feminists. In the early 1980s, this entrenchment of radical feminism with Liberalism and socialist Marxism began to change, with new scholarship and publications in the area of 'care ethics' from feminist authors such as Carol Gilligan and Nel Noddings. There was a shift from equality to relationality, and women's participation in caring relationships and roles in society. An early analysis of the theoretical framework of *care ethics* highlighted that caring was an alternative approach to moral reasoning to that of justice. Later theoretical explorations of *care ethics* examined political implications to care, particularly in a global context (Robinson, 2011). Care ethics became an alternative to what had been a focus on human rights or a Kantian framework for moral reasoning in educational and healthcare scholarship. This was achieved through the development of a narrative structure focusing on relationships, history and identity for moral understanding. In the early 1990s, nursing and midwifery scholarship embraced care ethics as an alternative to the dominant principlist moral reasoning framework developed in the early 1970s by American medical ethicists Beauchamp and Childress (2012). This emergence of an ethic of care within non-medical health professional scholarship enabled the development of subsequent feminist theoretical concepts – particularly relational autonomy, which will be discussed later in this chapter.

Few can agree about what and who encapsulates the third wave of feminism. The notion of a third wave of feminist theory began in the mid-1980s, at a time when there was the increased scholarly critique that postmodern feminist conceptions of womanhood were predominantly subjective (Gillis & Munford, 2006). Third-wave feminists identified to a degree with their second-wave 'sisters', but at the same time predicated their political and social position on distancing themselves from these earlier radical forms of and approaches to feminism (Dean, 2009). Characteristic of the third wave of feminism is the embracing of the traditional concepts of femininity, including the sexual power of women, and meshing this with traditional views of feminism. 'Lipstick', 'cybergirl' and 'Grrrl' feminisms are terms that detractors assign to the new generation of young feminists, 'many of who have no real clear sense of what feminist ideology, feminist praxis, feminist movement or feminist identity have meant across time and place' (Krolokke & Scott-Sorrensen, 2012: 15). Gamble (1998: 327) identifies the 'third wave' of feminist theory as being

> characterised by a desire to redress economic and racial inequality as well as 'women's issues' ... [and it] has been viewed with scepticism by many as merely a short-lived fashion rather than a genuine indication that women have reached the next stage in the feminist struggle.

It could be argued that the construction of third-wave feminist meaning has hinged on a series of simplifications and misconceptions about feminism, and as such has divided generations of feminists. In 1995, Rebecca Walker published *To Be Real: Telling the Truth and Changing the Face of Feminism*, which outlined a third-wave or explicitly feminist generation alternative to the feminism of previous generations. Leslie Heywood and Jennifer Drake's collection *Third Wave Agenda: Being Feminist, Doing Feminism* (1997), Ann Brooks' *Postfeminisms: Feminism, Cultural Theory and Cultural Forms* (1997), Natasha Walter's *The New Feminism* (1998), and Natasha Walter, Jennifer Baumgardner and Amy Richard's *Manifesta: Young Women, Feminism, and the Future* (2000) all emphasise the generational experience of being a woman in society after the gains of second-wave feminism. In Australia, key feminist writers representing this era include Melinda Tankard-Reist, Katrina George and Joanna Howe – all past or current members of third-wave feminist think-tank Women's Forum Australia.

It could be argued that third-wave feminists have not discarded the gains of radical feminism, but rather have incorporated certain features to create a hybrid of feminist meanings and apply these to more diverse contextual social, political and cultural circumstances. Claire Snyder (2008) argues that contemporary third-wave feminists make three important tactical moves in response to what they perceive as failings of their 'sisters' from the earlier radical feminist movement. For Snyder, third-wave feminists emphasise personal narratives that illustrate an intersectional and multi-perspective vision of feminism. This encapsulates much of the care ethics focus of second-wave feminists such as Noddings and Gilligan. Instead of presenting primarily a theoretical justification of feminism, third-wavers embrace social media to enhance their voice in matters of social, political and cultural injustices.

A significant difference between the second- and third-wave feminists is in response to the 'sex wars' prominent in the earlier radical period of feminism. Indeed, third-wave feminism focuses more on presenting an inclusive and non-judgemental approach to social and political activism (Snyder, 2008). The interpretation of mainstream feminism globally has included a questioning of how Western feminist theories have positively influenced postcolonial and developing world feminist practice (Valassopoulos, 2007). Essentially, third-wave feminism is inspired by a new global world order that is characterised by activism on both the local and global scale, and is inextricably linked to social media. Therefore, this new generation of feminists is not bound by particular theoretical or political positions, but rather by reviewing how globalisation and the redistribution of power in society inhibits liberation and creates oppression for women and other vulnerable members in society.

Difficulties in defining 'feminism'

In presenting the three waves of feminist theory and activism, the difficulty in identifying one definition of the term 'feminism' or describing what character-ises feminist theory becomes evident. The origin of the word *feminism* is quite modern. The term has French origins: it was used primarily as a word to describe the emancipation of women in Europe from the early 1890s. In May 1892, the first collective gathering of women to promote solidarity in the promotion of social and political equality was held in Paris. At this confer-ence, the term *feminisme* was juxtaposed with *masculinisme*, and subsequently became part of the Western political and social lexicon in the early twentieth century (Offen, 1988). Prominent US feminist bioethicist Professor Maggie Little (1996: 7) provides an academic definition of feminism and feminist theory as 'an attempt to uncover ways in which conceptions of gender distort people's views of the world and to articulate the ways in which these distortions, which are hurtful to all, are particularly constraining to women'. Advancing women's rights and equality has been the foundation of feminist activism and theory. Therefore, in understanding that feminist ethics is presenting a moral framework from a feminism perspective, it is also important to note that there exist many different kinds of feminism, and therefore differing characteristics to these definitions. In her book *Feminist Politics and Human Nature*, American philosopher Alison Jaggar (1983) presents four versions of feminism that provide a distinct view of the nature of oppression of women in society. These are Liberal, Marxist, radical and socialist feminist perspectives. Each version contributes distinct insights into the nature of the oppression of women. Liberal feminism focuses upon the lack of moral and legal rights for women in social institutions such as education, health and marriage. A Marxist view argues that there is an economic basis for women's oppression. Patriarchal influences on sex-gender systems form the foundation of radical feminism. Finally, the impact of class, race, age and gender under both a capitalist and patriarchal social system is the basis of Jaggar's definition of socialist feminism. Despite its historically marked origins, providing a contemporary academic definition of the term 'feminism' is problematic due to such diverse interpretations in the social, political and academic context over the last century.

It could be argued that the inability to present one singular definition of feminism or feminist theory has fostered open criticism and negative labelling of proponents of such activism, particular in Western socio-political cultures. One criticism is that feminism nurtures radical and militant women and is 'anti-men'. Another is that feminism has little relevance and meaning for the oppression of women in developing countries, non-English speaking cultures, and among indigenous populations. This area of multiculturalism and the application of feminism in non-Western cultures is worth exploring in more depth. Kathleen Heugh (2011) argues that the many NGO-sponsored education and health programs implemented in African cultures as a way to empower women have actually further alienated disadvantaged poor women in the Sub-Saharan region. She states that

> debates on transformation, equality and access need to have greater resonance in Africa. Cast from positions of either a western feminist maternalism or paternalism, they are equally disempowering of and interfere with the business of women in Africa. (2011: 101)

For Heugh, such Western feminist NGO-supported programs do not achieve the result of emancipation of women – ironically due to the majority of these programs being delivered by white, middle-class women teaching black women about marginalisation, oppression, racism and sexism. Warren (1989) affirms this perspective, arguing that for women living in developing countries, or from socio-economically oppressed races or cultures, a traditional conception of feminism must be expanded to represent a movement that not only aims to end sexist oppression, but *all* systems of oppression. Polish feminist Agnieszka Graff (2001) describes how a second- and third-wave narrative of feminism is not relevant in her cultural context by virtue of the absence of a recognisable women's movement in Poland prior to the fall of communism (Dean 2009). In critiquing Western feminist theory in an Asian cultural context, Bulbeck (2002) notes that the individual rights focus of Western feminism neglects the relational aspect of the woman living in a different kind of community. In non-Western cultures, where women may be relationally and culturally subordinated, to strive to be the agents of change through activism and disrupting personal and institutional power relations is virtually impossible for some women.

For many Western feminists, the needs and obligations of social collectivism and the influence of multiculturalism in non-Western cultures are often misrepresented and misunderstood. As American feminist writer Katha Pollitt states, 'You could say that multiculturalism demands respect for all cultural traditions, while feminism interrogates and challenges all cultural traditions'.

(cited in Moller-Okin, 1999: 27) Western feminists have vocally critiqued some developing world cultural practices, such as polygamy, female genital mutilation and multiparous births, as being disempowering for women. Despite such criticism, these same developed world feminists present minimal arguments about the need for economic and educational support, or tangible solutions, for women to be emancipated from these practices (Bulbeck, 2002). However, Indian academic Padma Anagol (2010) argues that elements of Western feminism have successfully been adapted in her culture, and that an 'indigenised' feminist framework has enabled oppressed women to have a voice in a traditional paternalism. She states that

> the term 'indigenous' does not refer to any search for 'authentic' or 'pure' origins but rather to the process by which Indian women's movements assimilated, negotiated, rejected or adapted aspects of western feminism whilst creating their own brand of Indian feminism (2010: 53).

It is of significance that, in response to recent targeted acts of sexual violence and physical bodily harm directed towards vulnerable women in India, it is young Indian women who are courageously presenting a unified voice through participation in public protests and engagement in social media to advance the legal rights of women in their country. This virtually based micro-activism – a key feature of third-wave feminism – went viral, and presented to the world an increased awareness of the socio-political injustices many women in India face on a daily basis.

'Relational autonomy' as a contemporary expression of feminist theory

This chapter has provided a historical analysis of feminism and discussion on applications of feminist theory in a non-Western construct. This next section will present a new concept featured in third-wave feminist theory – 'relational autonomy' – and will examine its application to healthcare ethics. A feminist approach to healthcare ethics has been increasingly prominent since the late 1980s. In a seminal article outlining such an approach, Little (1996) defines feminist bioethics as the examination of healthcare ethical issues from the perspective of feminist theory. Due to the diversity of feminist theoretical positions, a feminist approach to healthcare ethical reasoning can be, according to Little, at times a frustrating process. Some authors even argue that feminism has failed to contribute anything unique to healthcare ethics scholarship. Bioethicist Hilde Lindemann-Nelson (2000) argues that feminist contributions to healthcare ethics have remained predominantly a narrow critique, largely focused on androcentrism, paternalism and reproductive practices. She states:

> The point I want to make is that preoccupation with women's bodies, and especially women's reproductive health, leaves in place too many practices, institutions and assumptions of a sex-gender system that is biased in favour of men and this configures women as not only different, but deviant . . . our task is to come up with new theory, not to refine theories that leave everything exactly as it was. (2000: 495–6)

It is of some interest that the relatively new concept of 'relational autonomy' in contemporary third-wave feminist theory may provide a unique contribution to the scholarship of feminist healthcare ethics, and become one of these 'new' or 'refined' theories that Lindemann-Nelson advocates.

In 2000, feminist philosophers Catriona Mackenzie and Natalie Stoljar published an essay titled *Relational Autonomy*, in which they aimed to rehabil-itate the concept of respect for autonomy with an understanding of self in social and relational structures. For third-wave feminist scholars such as Mackenzie and Stoljar, being self-determining, self-sufficient and self-made is a masculine ideal that presents the ideal of self as an independent rather than relational being. Within a relational approach, autonomy emerges from within and, due to individuals being in relationships, their identity is shaped by social inter-actions in these interpersonal experiences. As Norton (2013: 297) suggests,

> feminists began to put forward alternative 'relational' models of autonomy, aiming to correct the atomism of traditional theories, and foreground the moral value of interpersonal relationships and the role they play in constitut-ing individual selves.

Essentially, relational models aimed at reconfiguring autonomy, which tradi-tionally had been central to the liberalism project; they wanted to present a new understanding that was sensitive to models of care, social interdependence and relationality. The relationally autonomous agent could be defined as a free, self-governing agent who is socially organised and defines basic value commitments in terms of interpersonal relationships and mutual dependencies (Christman, 2004).

Relational feminism emphasises women's rights in relation to others – women and men, principally defined by their nurturing and caring capacities.

This notion of relationality is a key focus of third-wave feminism, and differs significantly from the radical individualism of the second-wave theorists. Offen (1988: 136) highlights this contrast by stating that

> the individualist feminist tradition of argumentation emphasized more abstract concepts of individual human rights and celebrated the quest for personal independence (or autonomy) in all aspects of life, while downplaying, deprecating, or dismissing as insignificant all socially defined roles and minimizing discussion of sex-linked qualities or contributions, including childbearing and its attendant responsibilities.

Such contrast gives substantiation to Mackenzie's (2008) argument that relational autonomy is an umbrella term that covers a number of views. An agent's autonomy is inherently connected to their social-relational situation, which can vary according to situation and circumstance, and in a healthcare context, with progression of disease. Similarly, feminist ethical theories will question how the historical, social and relational context within which an agent is embedded impacts upon their capacity to be self-determining. Stoljar (2011) argues that feminist writing in this area emphasises the impact that gender, class, race, age and sexuality, and the role of social relationships and conditions, have upon these relationships. In application to clinical care, healthcare providers must be alert to social and relational conditions that may affect a patient's capacity for autonomous reasoning. In contemporary healthcare ethical literature, the notion of autonomy is synonymous with the concept of human rights and self-determination. The 'right' to ownership of one's body is the primary discourse in areas involving reproductive health and end-of-life decision-making. The concept of relational autonomy challenges the individualistic nature of ethical reasoning and decision-making in healthcare by arguing that no choice is made in isolation, but every decision will have communal implications.

A key reason why a healthcare environment has been the primary model for application of relational autonomy relates to the fact that, in such context, the ability to be self-determining and rational can be altered temporarily or permanently by illness, or by drug- and treatment-induced states. An extensive literature search on the topic of relational autonomy in healthcare ethics scholarship provides evidence of an increasing application in the area of psychology, informed consent, midwifery, female reproductive health and care of vulnerable members of the community – in particular, the aged, the mentally ill, and culturally and linguistically diverse populations. The midwifery model of care offers a unique clinical setting that would openly support integrating a relational autonomy approach within the healthcare context. Thachuk (2007) suggests that such an approach has profound implications on several relational levels, including that between woman and health professional (especially the midwife), and that between mother and unborn child. Similarly, changes in post-birth relationships between mother, child, partner and family have been explored in connection with relational autonomy and healthcare ethics research. In recent years, psychology research has focused on postnatal depression and relational autonomy (Goering, 2009). Goering argues that the well-being of new parents – in particular, a mother's capacity for autonomy – may be compromised by the myriad issues and experiences that come with childbirth. She states that

> a relational view of autonomy – attentive to the coercive effects of oppressive social norms and to the importance of developing autonomy competency, especially as related to self-trust – can improve our understanding of the situation of new parents and signal ways to cultivate and to better respect their autonomy (2009: 9).

Relationality, and not individualism, is therefore the key premise of this relational autonomy academic scholarship. It is a new and alternative approach to the traditional understanding of autonomy and ethical principlism in healthcare ethical reasoning.

In a review of multiculturalism and autonomy, Turoldo (2010) argues that relational autonomy is more morally acceptable, and indeed may present an analogous term of 'family autonomy' as being important in the provision of healthcare to culturally diverse groups. Earlier in this chapter, a critique of Western feminism in non-Western, developing world contexts was presented. It is possible that relational autonomy could be a unique approach to responding to the oppression of women in these cultures without imposing a Western feminist socio-political construct. Another scholarship area that explores relational autonomy in healthcare ethics literature is aged care. Perkins and colleagues (2012) studied relational autonomy in assisted aged care. Their research concluded that the provision of a relational autonomy model in assisted living

> provides a conceptual roadmap that can help us begin to deconstruct factors at multiple levels of social structure that interfere with resident autonomy and raise consciousness among policy makers, providers and family members regarding ways various social determinants shape residents' everyday lives (2012: 233).

Further implications of this research study relate to care of the person with dementia in an assisted living setting, which could be an important area for future feminist theoretical research and scholarship. Some ethicists argue that relational theories may not offer a fundamentally new approach to autonomy, in particular with application to healthcare ethics (Westlund, 2009). However, it is evident that contemporary third-wave feminist theorists and ethicists are challenging the traditional libertarian view of autonomy, and developing a dynamic and evolving shared meaning of autonomy in the provision of healthcare.

The application of relational autonomy in healthcare ethics can be explored through presenting a case study involving an unplanned pregnancy. Traditionally an area of radical feminist and liberation movement activism, the right of a woman to individual liberty, to be self-determining and have access to legal and safe termination of pregnancy treatment is a well-established field of contemporary feminist activism. Legal decisions involving abortion and other reproductive issues since the late 1960s have one principle that has been the primary force behind abortion access and rights for women: respect for autonomy. The belief that 'it is my body and my right' to terminate an unplanned pregnancy became the mantra, and encapsulated a radical notion of autonomy and reproductive rights that was bereft of any perception of transcendent moral responsibility or accountability to the others, including the unborn foetus. Informed consent was based on the ability to make an individual choice relative to the unplanned or unwanted pregnancy. However, such consent in the liberal tradition does not ensure that the context in which the choices have been made are optimal for ensuring true capacity for autonomy (Laufer-Ukeles, 2011). Immediately, the woman is relational to her unborn embryo or foetus, even if it is an unplanned or unwanted pregnancy. Conception was also achieved through sexual intercourse, which is a relational activity. The woman would also be in a social context, with family and/or friends who may influence her decision-making in this scenario.

Visiting a health professional for more information to morally and practically reason her final choice, the pregnant woman also engages other persons into her sphere of decision-making. Even a consideration of the future interests of self and any yet-to-be conceived children may impact a woman's decision in this given scenario. Therefore, under a normative ethical framework of relational autonomy, the focus on individualism and informed consent is challenged, as such extended relationships are deemed necessary to support the woman's autonomous choice – whatever that may be. As Laufer-Ukeles suggests:

> Relational autonomy seeks to create a framework for enhancing and optimiz-
> ing autonomous decision making through dialogue and explicit recognition
> of social and contextual pressures involved in choice. (2011: 611)

The woman does not make her decision regarding her unplanned pregnancy in a 'moral reasoning silo', as the liberal and individualistic notion of autonomy would support. Importantly, relational autonomy acknowledges that coercive factors from her relationships impact on a woman's decision-making about an unplanned pregnancy – something that the liberal tradition of consent does not. As most reproductive choices are made in non-emergency situations, the ability to maximise a woman's autonomy to ensure that her final choice is one that is genuine, weighs up all options and presents with reference to her relationships with others is the ideal. A relational autonomy model of consent for a woman seeking a termination of pregnancy would result in a joint decision-making dialogue, emphasise the importance of broad values and interests not only for the woman, ensure that there is an understanding of the long-term relational impact of such a decision and, finally, acknowledge the complex social forces and values that will influence the woman's final decision.

Conclusion

By undertaking a historical review of the foundations of feminism and feminist theory, it is evident that a single definition of these terms, and application into a societal and cultural context, are challenging. Through a review of some of the characteristics of each historical period – in particular, the review of contemporary understanding of feminism 'waves' – it is possible to identify some congruencies in theoretical foundations and, at the same time, the adaptation that feminism has made within a changing and divergent socio-political context. Constituting a relatively under-researched framework in bioethics, feminism and feminist theory have significant value for advocating and advancing the rights of women and other vulnerable members of society in the healthcare context. The exploration of relational autonomy, and its application in morally uncertain situations in healthcare, represent a contemporary and exciting new foray for feminist healthcare ethics research. This chapter has provided a brief overview of these concepts. It is hoped that, in the future, healthcare professionals will be increasingly open and able to engage actively with contemporary feminist theory in assisting moral reasoning in the care of the vulnerable members of society.

Reflective exercises

10.1 In this chapter, a historical timeline has been presented to help us explore feminist theory. Map out your own timeline, and present some of the key social, cultural and political factors that have shaped each moment in the timeline.

10.2 Simone de Beauvoir's primary thesis in *The Second Sex* was that men fundamentally oppress women by characterising them, on every level, as the 'Other' – or the second and subordinate sex to men. For de Beauvoir, defining woman exclusively as the 'Other' sex, denies her humanity.

- With relation to the three waves of feminism presented in the chapter, has there been an evolution of this original feminist premise asserted by de Beauvoir? If so, what may be some contributing factors?
- Review this statement with relation to contemporary healthcare provision in your clinical practice. Are there any examples where this statement may be evident? What are some of the cultural, social or political factors that may be influential in this occurrence?

10.3 Grainger argues that feminism is predominantly a Western construct, and its influence in non-Western cultures may be viewed as tenuous. Do you agree or disagree with this assertion? What are the key arguments to strengthen your position?

10.4 As an example of contemporary feminist thought in the provision of healthcare, Grainger presents the concept of relational autonomy.

- What are some of the key elements to this concept, and how does it differ from the traditional notion of autonomy in healthcare delivery?
- In this chapter, relational autonomy has been presented in relation to decision-making for a woman with an unplanned pregnancy. What are some other areas in healthcare provision where this notion of relational autonomy could be applied? What may be some of the benefits or limitations of such a framework for ethical decision-making for both the patient/client and the healthcare professional?

References

Anagol. P. (2010). Feminist inheritances and foremothers: The beginnings of feminism in modern India. *Women's History Review*, 19(4): 523–46.

Beauchamp, T. L. & Childress, J. F. (2013). *Principles of biomedical ethics* (7th ed.). New York: Oxford University Press.

Bowden, P. & Mummery, J. (2009). *Understanding feminism*. Stocksfield (UK): Acumen.

Brooks, A. (1997). *Postfeminisms: Feminism, cultural theory and cultural forms*. New York: Routledge.

Bulbeck, C. (2002). Asian perspectives on Western feminism: Interrogating the assumption. *China Report*, 38(2): 179–91.

Christman, J. (2004). Relational autonomy, liberal individualism and the social constitution of selves. *Philosophical Studies*, 117: 143–64.

Coole, D. (1988). *Women in political theory: From ancient misogyny to contemporary feminism*. Loughborough: Harvester Wheatsheaf.

Dean, J. (2009). Who's afraid of third wave feminism? On the uses of the 'third wave' in British feminist politics. *International Feminist Journal of Politics*, 11(3): 334–52.

de Beauvoir, S. (1952). *The second sex*. New York: Vintage.

Friedan, B. (1963). *The feminine mystique*. New York: W.W. Norton.

Gamble, S. (1998). *The Routledge companion to feminism and postfeminism*. London: Routledge.

Gillis, S. & Munford, R. (2006). Genealogies and generations: The politics and praxis of third wave feminism. *Women's History Review*, 13(2): 165–82.

Gluck, S. B. (1988). *Rosie the Riveter revisited: Women, the war and social change*. New York: Penguin.

Goering, S. (2009). Postnatal reproductive autonomy: Promoting relational autonomy and self-trust in patients. *Bioethics*, 23(1): 9–19.

Graff, A. (2001). *World without women*. Warsaw: WAB.

Greer, G. (1970). *The female eunuch*. London: Harper Perennial.

Heugh, K. (2011). Discourses from without, discourses from within: Women, feminism and voice in Africa. *Current Issues in Language and Planning*, 12(1): 89–104.

Heywood, L. & Drake, J. (1997). *Third wave agenda: Being feminist, doing feminism*. Minneapolis, MN: University of Minnesota Press.

Howie, G. & Tauchert, A. (2007). Feminist dissonance: The logic of late feminism. In S. Gillis, G. Howie & R. Munford (eds), *Third wave feminism: A critical exploration* (2nd ed.). New York: Palgrave Macmillan.

Jaggar, A. (1983). *Feminist politics and human nature*. Oxford: Rowman and Littlefield.

Krolokke, C. & Scott-Sorensen, A. (2012). *Gender communication theories and analyses: From silence to performance.* Thousand Oaks, CA: Sage.

Laufer-Ukeles, P. (2011). Reproductive choices and informed consent: Fetal interests, women's identity and relational autonomy. *American Journal of Law and Medicine,* 37(4): 687–9.

Lindemann-Nelson, H. (2000). Feminist bioethics: Where we've been, where we's going. *Metaphysiology,* 31(5): 492–508.

Little, M. (1996). Why a feminist approach to bioethics? *Kennedy Institute of Ethics Journal,* 6(1): 1–18.

Mackenzie, C. (2008). Relational autonomy, normative authority and perfectionism. *Journal of Social Philosophy,* 39(4): 512–33.

Mackenzie, C. & Stoljar, N. (2000). *Relational autonomy: Feminist perspectives on autonomy, agency and the social self.* Oxford: Oxford University Press.

Mill, J. S. (1869). *The subjection of women.* London: Longmans, Green, Reader & Dyer.

Millett, K. (1969). *Sexual politics.* New York: Doubleday.

Mitchell, J. (1974). *Psychoanalysis and feminism: Freud, Reich, Laing and women.* New York: Random House.

Moller-Okin, S. (1999). *Is multiculturalism bad for women?* Princeton, NJ: Princeton University Press.

Norton, B. M. (2013). Emma Courtney, feminist ethics and the problem of autonomy. *The Eighteenth Century,* 54(3): 297–315.

Offen, K. (1988). Defining feminism: A comparative historical approach. *Signs,* 14(1): 119–57.

Perkins, M. M., Ball, M. M., Whittington, F. J. & Hollingsworth, C. (2012). Relational autonomy in assisted living: A focus on diverse care settings for older adults. *Journal of Ageing Studies,* 26: 214–25.

Robinson, F. (2011). *The ethics of care: A feminist approach to human security.* Philadelphia, PA: Temple University Press.

Snyder, R. C. (2008). What is third-wave feminism? A new directions essay. *Journal of Women in Culture and Society,* 34(1): 175–96.

Stoljar, N. (2011). Autonomy, informed consent and relational conceptions of autonomy. *Journal of Medicine and Philosophy,* 36: 375–84.

Thachuk, A. (2007). Midwifery, informed choice, and reproductive autonomy: A relational approach. *Feminism & Psychology,* 17(1): 39–56.

Turoldo, F. (2010). Relational autonomy and multiculturalism. *Cambridge Quarterly of Health Care Ethics,* 19: 542–9.

Valassopoulos, A. (2007). 'Also I wanted so much to leave for the West': Postcolonial feminism rides the third wave. In S. Gillis, G. Howie & R. Munford (eds), *Third wave feminism: A critical exploration* (2nd ed.). New York: Palgrave Macmillan.

Vanstone, A. (2002). Australian suffragettes, *Australian Story*, ABC TV. Retrieved 20 February 2014 from <http://australia.gov.au/about-australia/australian-story/austn-suffragettes>.

Walker, R. (1995). *To be real: Telling the truth and changing the face of feminism*. London: Anchor Books.

Walter, N. (1998). *The new feminism*. London: Virago.

Walter, N., Baumgardner, J. & Richard, A. (2000). *Manifesta:*

Young women, feminism and the future. New York: Farrar, Straus and Giroux.

Warren, K. (1989). Reconceiving feminism. *Social Philosophy Today*, 2: 135–46.

Westlund, A. C. (2009). Rethinking relational autonomy, *Hypatia*, 24(4): 26–49.

Wollstonecraft, M. (1995 [1792]). *A vindication of the rights of women*. Cambridge: Cambridge University Press.

11 Conscience and the healthcare professional

Brigid McKenna

If all the world hated you and believed you wicked,
while your own conscience approved of you and absolved
you from guilt, you would not be without friends.

– Charlotte Brontë, *Jane Eyre*

Conscience is widely recognised as a universal, yet highly personal, human phenomenon. In recent times, however, the role of conscience in public and professional life has increasingly been challenged. This chapter explores whether conscience is indeed the 'friend' or 'foe' of healthcare professionals and all those who seek their services. It proposes a definition of conscience that is grounded in traditional ethics, and introduces the reader to the concept and practice of conscientious objection. This is followed by an analysis of challenges to the legitimacy of conscientious objection in a contemporary healthcare system, and a discussion of how the case for or against conscientious objection ultimately depends on competing models of healthcare and professionalism. The chapter concludes with proposals for how conscientious objection might best be accommodated in a contemporary healthcare setting.

What is conscience?

Most people – including most scholars – presume that conscience exists, and that its function is to alert us to a potential conflict between values and to indicate which values should guide our choices (Morton & Kirkwood, 2009). Nevertheless, many of the disputes about the role of conscience in healthcare proceed on the basis of differing definitions of conscience (Lawrence & Curlin, 2007; Morton & Kirkwood, 2009; Sulmasy, 2008).

For this reason, it is important to define clearly both what conscience *is* and what it *is not*.

Conscience is not a little voice, distinct from our own reasoning, that urges us towards a particular course of action or admonishes us for past transgressions. It is certainly not two little voices – often figuratively depicted as an angel and a devil – that whisper conflicting advice in our ear and fight for our soul. Conscience is not separate and outside of us, or even separate but within us. Conscience is *integral to who we are as human persons*. Rather than being a distinct faculty, conscience engages our whole person. In this regard, conscience is not something that we possess, but something that we *do*: the human mind thinking practically towards good choices (Fisher, 2012)

Conscience is also much more than an intuitive moral sense or a feeling. The judgements of conscience may involve or be associated with emotions (for example, satisfaction, guilt, apprehension, repugnance, calm), but they are ultimately *based in reason* and consequently, able to be explained and challenged. Conscience is an intellectual activity that arises in particular ethical deliberations. It involves thinking about fundamental ethical principles and how they apply to a concrete situation; this ultimately results in a rational decision about what ought to be done or not done in a particular situation. In this regard, Sulmasy (2008: 138) defines conscience as having two interrelated parts:

- a commitment to morality itself, to acting and choosing morally according to the best of one's ability, and
- the activity of judging that an act one has done or about which one is deliberating would violate that commitment.

Conscience can also be understood as the guardian of individual authenticity and integrity (Morton & Kirkwood, 2009). Because they alert an individual to potential or past violations of personal values, judgements of conscience 'constitute the central bases of individuals' moral integrity; they define who, at least morally speaking, the individual is, what she stands for, what is the central moral core of her character' (Brock, 2008: 189).

However, this does not mean that judgements of conscience will always be morally right. Conscience is not infallible: people can choose conscientiously and wrongly as a result of one or more of the following: ignorance of important facts, moral rules, or even one's own moral commitments; faulty moral reasoning; emotional imbalance; or poor judgement (Sulmasy, 2008). This possibility of objective moral error gives rise to the personal and professional duty to both *inform* and *form* our conscience. It does not, however, detract from the further duty to always follow the judgements of our conscience: if conscience is our best judgement about what ought or ought not be done in a particular situation, personal integrity demands that we follow its dictates (Laabs, 2009; Pellegrino, 2002).

Some authors distinguish between a 'religious' and a 'secular' conscience (e.g. Dickens & Cook, 2000). Certainly, while fundamental moral commitments, principles, laws or values will often be based in religious belief, this is not always – and need not always be – the case. Davis, Schrader and Belcheir (2012) found that conscientious objection and moral distress were more likely to affect nurses whose ethical beliefs were most influenced by their religious beliefs than nurses whose ethical beliefs were influenced by family values, life and work experience, political views or the professional code of ethics. By contrast, a survey of medical students conducted by Strickland (2012) found that a greater percentage of conscientious objections were for non-religious reasons than religious ones, suggesting that non-religious beliefs can be just as firmly held and as central to a person's moral life as religious beliefs. It makes little sense, however, to talk of 'religious' and 'secular' consciences as if they are somehow different. Even if the content of conscience (the fundamental moral commitments) differs from person to person, the basic function of conscience (to apply fundamental moral commitments to concrete situations) and its effect on each person are the same (Morton & Kirkwood, 2009; Sulmasy, 2008).

What is the role of conscience in healthcare?

It is traditionally perceived, and still widely understood, that healthcare is a moral or ethical activity, and not merely a technical one. As well as determining the strictly therapeutic or clinical merit of a particular course of action, healthcare professionals are frequently required to determine whether or not an action is good or bad, right or wrong in an ethical sense. In view of the fact that they provide healthcare to people, and not only to their bodies, healthcare professionals' decisions will regularly be 'conscientious decisions', which attempt to align their actions towards patients/clients with their own fundamental moral commitments. This is not to say that acting in accordance with conscience is always easy. There are numerous healthcare situations where doing the right thing can be extremely difficult, such as telling the truth about a bad prognosis, exposing incompetent or unethical colleagues and practices, or challenging organisational short-fallings in staffing levels or other cost-containment measures. These situations call for 'moral courage' in addition to conscientious decision-making (Gallagher, 2010; Murray, 2010).

Essentially, conscience is used (or 'exercised') by healthcare professionals when they choose to avoid doing what is apparently evil or engage in doing what is apparently good (Murphy & Genuis, 2013). However, most of the academic discussion and public controversy about the role of conscience in healthcare concerns the former situation, and what is commonly referred to as *conscientious objection*. A conscientious objection is the refusal to act against one's moral convictions. In the healthcare setting, conscientious objection is a healthcare professional's refusal to 'follow a specified course of action requested by a patient, or expected by general practice guidelines, on the basis of a conflict with personal values, beliefs or morals' (Morton & Kirkwood, 2009: 356). The action in question is usually legal and professionally acceptable, but morally unacceptable to the healthcare professional. Indeed, an authentic act of conscientious objection must be based upon deeply held moral convictions, and not upon personal whim, aesthetics, inconvenience or prejudice. Furthermore, the focus of conscientious objection should always be upon a type of procedure or service, and never upon a particular 'type' of patient or client. Healthcare professionals should never discriminate against a person on medically irrelevant grounds such as race, religion, sex, age or nationality (Magelssen, 2012).

At least in Western societies, increasing cultural, religious and moral pluralism could make conscientious objection a more commonplace characteristic of healthcare practice (Magelssen, 2012). This is especially likely as medical knowledge is increasingly used for purposes other than treating disease (Sulmasy, 2008). The circle of healthcare professionals engaging in conscientious objection could include, among others, the 'pro-life' theatre nurse who refuses to assist with abortions, the Catholic pharmacist who refuses to dispense oral contraceptives, the child health nurse who refuses to provide information and referral for infant circumcision or the Jewish doctor who refuses to withdraw life-prolonging treatment.

Some commentators emphasise that the *provision* of ethically controversial medical services, such as abortion, can also be conscience based, and argue that respect for conscience requires accommodation of commitment to their delivery as well as refusal to participate (Dickens & Cook, 2011; Harris, 2012). This raises the question, however, of whether or not it is possible for opposing claims (such as one 'for' and the other 'against' participation in abortion) to be equally conscientious and equally deserving of respect. This position also overlooks the significant moral difference between preventing someone from doing what they believe to be good and forcing someone to do what they believe to be wrong (Murphy & Genuis, 2013).

The ability of a healthcare professional to engage in conscientious objection is widely regarded as an expression of the natural or basic human right to freedom of conscience. Article 18(1) of the United Nations International Covenant on Civil and Political Rights provides that: 'Everyone shall have the right to freedom of thought, conscience and religion ... [and] to manifest his religion or belief in worship, observance, practice and teaching.' However, freedom of conscience is not absolute. Article 18(3) provides that: 'Freedom to manifest one's religion or beliefs may be subject only to such limitations as ... are necessary to protect public safety, order, health, or morals or the fundamental rights and freedoms of others.' Clearly, different interpretations of Article 18(3) will have a significant influence upon legal provisions for conscientious objection in healthcare.

Statements endorsing conscientious objection and listing circumstances in which it might be expressed are also reflected in most healthcare professional codes of ethics and related position statements (e.g. see Nursing and Midwifery Board of Australia, 2008, Value Statement 1; Australian Nursing Federation, 2011; Australian Medical Council, 2009, 2.4.6; Australian Medical Association, 2013; Pharmacy Board of Australia, 2010, 2.4). Laws covering freedom of conscience or the right to claim conscientious objection – so called 'conscience clauses' – are also found in all Australian states and many overseas jurisdictions. These usually relate to termination of pregnancy, and provide that no person is under a duty – whether by contract, statutory or other legal requirement – to perform a termination to which they have a conscientious objection (O'Rourke, De Crespigny & Pyman, 2013).

The case for freedom of conscience for healthcare professionals

Until recently, a healthcare professional's right to freedom of conscience was widely accepted, and conscientious objection was rarely questioned. Indeed, outside of sectors of academia and certain special-interest groups, it is still largely expected that healthcare professionals are people 'of conscience', and that this is especially the case when they are at work. This view recognises that the exercise of conscience by healthcare professionals has real benefits for both practitioners and their patients. Birchley (2011: 16) describes these benefits as follows:

> It provides a mental space where practitioners can reflect upon their experiences and improve their practice; heeding conscience may allow them to remain sensitive to both their own and their patients' needs; conscience provides a voice to moral objection that is independent of dominant mores and hierarchy and an instant alarm when events begin rapidly to outpace the speed with which we can consider them. By fostering and respecting it, engaging with and interrogating its judgments, it will benefit practice and practitioners alike.

At the same time, there is growing recognition – particularly within the nursing profession – that *restrictions* upon freedom of conscience that result in violations of one's moral integrity can lead to physical and mental symptoms consistent with 'moral distress'. Moral distress involves feelings of anger, anxiety, guilt, sorrow, frustration and helplessness, which can have a significant effect on self-esteem, self-respect, patient care, job satisfaction and burnout (Birchley, 2011; Davis, Schrader & Belcheir, 2009; Morton & Kirkwood, 2009). It is generally acknowledged as the outcome where one knows the ethically correct action to take but feels powerless to take that action (Epstein & Delgado, 2010). In this regard, workplace environments in which non-compliance with 'orders' may be a dismissible offence pose significant risks for nurses who refuse to participate in certain medical procedures or organisational processes (Dickens & Cook, 2000). Often, it will be far easier to 'silently' conscientiously object 'by sidestepping a particular patient assignment, changing shifts, declining to work in a particular ward or area, or taking a "sick day" off work' (Johnstone, 2009: Ch. 13). Unfortunately, environments where there is poor communication and explanation of decisions made by doctors and other team members may lead to conflicts of conscience, and precipitate unnecessary moral distress for nurses (Corley, 2002). For example, without explanation of the reasons behind a doctor's order to withdraw a life-sustaining treatment, a nurse might mistakenly think that they have been asked to participate in euthanasia by omission, when the doctor's intention is simply to cease treatment which has become medically futile or overly burdensome for the patient.

Persistently acting against one's conscience can also result in desensitisation of the conscience. Conscience has a motivating function: the infliction of guilt, remorse and distress when we act against our core values provides a warning and motivation to realign our choices with our values. However, if the ethical conflict causing distress is not resolved, there is a risk that practitioners will eventually learn to ignore the cautionary and motivating effects of conscience, and in so doing, weaken their capacity for ethical decision-making (Lawrence & Curlin, 2007; Morton & Kirkwood, 2009). This is an important reason why it is generally problematic to expect healthcare professionals to be 'people of conscience', but demand that they ignore their consciences in certain circumstances. This position is echoed by Laabs (2009: 12) in reference in nursing:

> To expect nurses to set aside their conscience is to endorse an unfeasible stance of value neutrality toward the moral work of nursing, a perilous stance that risks indifference toward patients who have placed their lives in the hands of persons they count on to care for and about them.

'Objections' to conscientious objection

If we accept that conscientious objection benefits healthcare professionals and, in a secondary way, confers general benefits to patients, what can be said about situations where the conscientious refusal of particular medical services causes significant inconvenience, and possibly even harm, to the person making the request?

In 2009, the media (Gregory, 2009; Mayoh, 2009) reported that a Catholic pharmacist in regional New South Wales was refusing to sell the oral contraceptive pill, the morning-after pill and condoms because of his religious and moral beliefs. The pharmacist told the media:

> When I dispense an oral contraceptive pill I will ask the lady to sit at our counselling desk where I explain that there is a leaflet in the box regarding our pharmacy policy on the pill. It explains that I accept the teachings of the Catholic Church against the use of artificial contraception, and asks the lady to respect my view on the use of artificial contraception and have it filled elsewhere next time if it is being taken for contraceptive purposes.

Opinions were divided over whether or not this pharmacist was meeting his 'professional' obligations and duty of care to his clients. A representative from Family Planning NSW was reported as saying that contraceptive options should not be taken away by a healthcare professional's personal beliefs, while a spokesman for the Pharmacy Guild of Australia said that pharmacists, like anyone, were entitled to hold ethical, religious or moral views, and that individual pharmacies were entitled to sell, or not sell, any product or medication they liked.

The spokesman also pointed out that the town had a number of pharmacies where people could go for contraceptive and morning-after pills, and that condoms were freely available outside of pharmacies. But what if the objecting pharmacist were the only pharmacist in town? Would they still be justified in their conscientious refusal to supply a legally available, prescribed medication? Should there be limits to the scope and practice of conscientious objection?

This example demonstrates how the role of conscience and, more specifically, the 'right' of healthcare professionals to exercise conscientious objection, has become a 'hot-button' topic in modern healthcare practice, especially with its strong emphasis on respect for patient autonomy.

Reflecting upon the medical profession, Charo (2005: 2473) argues that doctors cannot claim an 'absolute' right to conscientious objection to the provision of particular medical services, so long as the state gives these professionals the exclusive right to offer such services:

> By granting a monopoly, (states) turn the profession into a kind of public utility obligated to provide service to all who seek it. Claiming an unfettered right to personal autonomy while holding monopolistic control over a public good constitutes an abuse of the public trust . . .

Similar arguments distinguish between those healthcare professionals who work within publicly funded systems and those who work in privately funded systems. Savulescu (2006: 296) concedes that doctors in private elective medicine have 'more liberty to offer the service of their choice based upon their values', provided that they inform their patients of relevant alternatives. As 'public servants', however, doctors 'must act in the public interest, not their own' (2006: 297). Similar arguments are also extended to publicly funded religious healthcare institutions and services (Dickens, 2009).

One response to this position is that it is not individual healthcare professionals, but rather the healthcare *profession*, that holds a publicly instituted and legal monopoly to provide healthcare. Unless the entire profession refused to provide a particular service, the presence of monopolistic control over a public good is not a compelling reason for overriding the professional conscience of individual practitioners (Kaczor, 2012).

Savulescu (2006), however, takes his position against conscientious objection even further. He regards the duty to provide legal services as a defining 'commitment' for doctors. By his account, there is simply no place for conscientious objection that compromises the quality, efficiency or equitable distribution of a health service, such as when patients are left to shop around for a doctor who will provide the service, or when other less informed or resourceful patients will simply miss out on a service to which they are legally entitled. Savulescu states unequivocally that: 'If people are not prepared to offer legally permitted, efficient, and beneficial care to a patient because it conflicts with their values, they should not be doctors.' (2006: 294) Although his focus here is upon doctors, he gives no indication as to why this position should not also apply to other healthcare professionals.

Other commentators argue that conscientious refusal to provide particular services should exclude practitioners from working in certain areas – for example, the conscientious refusal to provide pregnancy termination services should be a valid reason for doctors (and, by extension, other healthcare professionals) to avoid the practice of modern perinatal medicine (Blustein & Fleischman, 1995). Cantor (2009) writes: 'As the gatekeepers to medicine, physicians and other health providers have an obligation to choose specialties that are not moral minefields for them. Qualms about abortion, sterilization, and birth control? Do not practice women's health.' (1484)

However, if we accept that personal conscience is dynamic and evolving, an obvious response to this line of reasoning is that it is not always possible for budding healthcare professionals to anticipate future conflicts of conscience in general or speciality practice. A person entering an undergraduate nursing program or medical school, perhaps as young as 18 years of age, might not possess sufficient life experience to have a fully developed and stable conscience. More specifically,

> only through the experience of practicing and confronting conflicts can a practitioner discover which personal values conflict with his or her professional duties, and determine whether those conflicts are the result of erroneous beliefs or not (Morton & Kirkwood, 2009: 360–1).

If we want healthcare professionals to be people 'of conscience' who bring their values to work, it is inevitable that conflicts of values will arise between practitioners and patients. In this regard, Morton and Kirkwood (2009: 360–1) propose that:

> It is more important that we recognize this as a feature of being a conscientious member of society and facilitate the development of skills for addressing these issues, than that we attempt the impossible feat of screening out every person with an offending view. Such an extreme policy might result in very few, if any,

people qualifying for practice, or worse, only allow those individuals without a sensitive conscience to practice.

Excluding – or, at the very least, discouraging – people with particular moral viewpoints from entering healthcare professions or specialties would also unjustly discriminate against people who hold a religious or philosophical 'pro-life' perspective. Ironically, this could result in restrictions upon patient choice of the type of person from whom they wish to receive healthcare.

A third reason to argue against the legitimacy of conscientious objection in healthcare is based upon the view that healthcare professionals have an obligation to place patient interests (and autonomy) before their own personal interests (and autonomy). When they enter a healthcare 'profession', individual practitioners 'profess' to elevate patient interests above personal interests. This makes them willing to risk their own well-being for the good of their patients, such as by exposing themselves to dangerous diseases in the course of treating patients. If they are willing to sacrifice their lives, surely they should also be prepared to sacrifice their moral integrity for the good of their patients (Dickens, 2009).

However, critics of this position argue that healthcare professionals do not have an absolute duty to always place patient interests above their own, and that there is an important distinction between healthcare professionals risking harm to themselves (such as by treating patients during an outbreak of an infectious disease) and certainly harming oneself (for example, by refusing any payment for services). By their account, acting against one's conscience, such as when one is compelled to violate a deeply held belief in the inviolability of human life by performing or assisting with a termination of pregnancy, falls into the second category of 'certain harm' to a healthcare professional's moral integrity (Kaczor, 2012; Wicclair, 2008).

It should also be pointed out that conscientious objection often concerns procedures (abortion, sterilisation, circumcision, euthanasia, in-vitro fertilisation) that fall outside of the scope of the traditional view that healthcare is for healing. This is sometimes also expressed as a distinction between medical care and non-medical care that uses medical services (Charo, 2005). By this account, the 'interests of patients' that a healthcare professional would be required to put above their own personal interests would be limited to the restoration of health, and likely extended to the prevention of illness (Wicclair, 2008). In the specific case of abortion, a conscientious objector is also likely to regard the foetus as a second 'patient', with 'interests' of their own.

Healthcare professionals or healthcare providers?

While some disagreements over the role assigned to professional conscience in healthcare can be traced back to different understandings of what conscience is, others are fundamentally based in competing conceptions or models of healthcare, and whether practitioners are viewed as healthcare 'providers' or healthcare 'professionals'.

A model of healthcare that emphasises the moral agency of the practitioner and, more often than not, prioritises traditional goals of healing, generally affirms and supports conscientious objection by healthcare practitioners. However, a model of healthcare that emphasises the moral agency of the patient/client and prioritises the provision of requested health services generally undermines and opposes the legitimacy of conscientious objection.

The former emphasises professional autonomy and the service of healing; the latter emphasises patient autonomy and service provision. While one is criticised for 'violating the right of adults to self-determination', the other is criticised for 'diminishing the moral agency and responsibility of physicians by making them mere technicians or vendors of health care goods' (Curlin et al., 2007: 599). In order to substantively address the role of conscience in health care, we are ultimately faced with questions of whether, or to what extent, medical decision-making should lie with the healthcare professional or with the patient, and whether the ends and goals of healthcare should be defined by healthcare professionals, or by patients, social convention and the law (Pellegrino, 2002).

What, then, is the practical and ethical way forward? One study found that most doctors seek a balance between these extremes, which involves both full disclosure of the practitioner's relevant conscientious views, with disclosure of all information and open dialogue about the options at hand. In this way they conform to

> models for the doctor–patient relationship that retain the moral agency of both the physician and the patient by encouraging them to engage in a dialogue and negotiate mutually acceptable accommodations that do not require either of the parties to violate their own convictions (Curlin et al., 2007: 599).

A further controversy is whether or not a healthcare professional with a conscientious objection to a requested treatment is obliged to refer the patient to receive the controversial treatment from another practitioner. On this issue, professional codes of practice, law and ethical opinion are divided.

Many ethicists regard the provision of a referral as a minimal obligation for conscientious objectors (Cantor & Baum, 2004; Dickens & Cook, 2000; Savulescu, 2006). Charo (2005) argues that because acts of conscience are usually accompanied by a 'willingness to pay some price', healthcare professionals should at least accept a 'collective obligation', which ensures that 'a genuine system for counselling and referring patients is in place, so that every patient can act according to his or her own conscience just as readily as the professional can' (Charo, 2005: 2471). More precisely, Savulescu (2006: 296) argues that: 'Any would-be conscientious objector must ensure that patients know about and receive care that they are entitled to from another professional in a timely manner that does not compromise their access to care.' By this account, it is unacceptable to leave patients to fend for themselves at the cost of their health or other interests (Dickens & Cook, 2000).

Advocates of an obligation to refer tend, however, to understate the personal implications of referral for conscientious objectors. They think it is enough that, following referral, objectors usually have no further part to play in discussions between the patient and the healthcare professional who has received the referral, or any further financial or other benefits to reap (Dickens, 2009). For many conscientious objectors, though, the simple act of referral is held to be morally unacceptable cooperation in the wrongdoing of others; in this sense, referral renders them complicit in the objectionable procedure. Indeed, determining whether one is complicit in such wrongdoing is itself a judgement of conscience, with important implications for the practitioner. Murphy and Genuis (2013: 349–50) explain the significance of complicity as follows:

> There appears to be something about complicity in wrongdoing that triggers an instinctive and profound sense of abhorrence. A sense of uncleanness, taint, or shame arising from complicity in wrongdoing – even if it is coerced – is the natural response of the human person to something fundamentally opposed to his/her nature and dignity.

Magelssen (2012) describes any participation in the causal chain leading to the disputed treatment – such as circumstances where an objecting practitioner is required to arrange referral to another doctor – as a 'serious violation' of moral integrity. However, he distinguishes this from a lesser sense of 'referral', where all that is required is informing the patient about practitioners who can assist them with their request. In some jurisdictions, attempts have been made to legislate in accordance with this distinction.

In Victoria, if a woman requests a registered health practitioner to advise on a proposed abortion, or to perform, direct, authorise or supervise an abortion for that woman, and the practitioner has a conscientious objection to abortion, the practitioner is legally obligated to both inform the woman that the practitioner has a conscientious objection to abortion and refer the woman to another registered health practitioner in the same regulated health profession who the practitioner knows does not have a conscientious objection to abortion (*Abortion Law Reform Act 2008*, s 8(1)).

Supporters of the law argue that the 'obligation to refer' is necessary to protect patients from being deprived of the right to choose abortion and other lawful treatments according to their conscience, by unknowingly seeing a practitioner who either refuses to offer abortions or presents information in a way that deprives the patient of choice (O'Rourke, De Crespigny & Pyman, 2013). They cite legal opinion that the law 'may be complied with if a doctor with a conscientious objection simply refers his or her patient to a public hospital or to a recognised independent pregnancy service' (Burnside, cited in O'Rourke, De Crespigny & Pyman, 2013: 108).

This law is, however, surrounded by confusion and controversy. It goes well beyond existing professional guidelines, which state that a conscientious objector must not 'impede access to treatments that are legal' but do *not* require referral to a non-objecting practitioner (Australian Medical Council, 2009, 2.4.6; Australian Medical Association, 2013). The insertion of an active duty to refer places Victorian practitioners who conscientiously object to abortion in all, or even only some, circumstances in a difficult position, as many regard 'referral' for a medical procedure as a recommendation of the procedure. They take the view that even though the law does not require conscientious objectors to refer directly to an abortion provider, if a patient has made a choice to have an abortion, a referral to a non-objecting practitioner will in all likelihood result in an abortion being obtained. Many conscientious objectors see even this type of referral as facilitating the abortion, making them morally complicit in the objectionable act (Smith, 2013). As recently as 2013, a Victorian general practitioner was investigated after conscientiously refusing to refer a woman who was seeking a sex-selection abortion at 19 weeks' gestation to a non-objecting practitioner (Rolfe, 2013).

Tonti-Filippini (2013) reports the Victorian law is already forcing some conscientious health practitioners out of particular areas of healthcare practice, or causing them to abandon practice altogether. This is, he says, obviously discriminatory for practitioners who respect the right to life of the unborn, as well as unnecessary in view of the fact that abortion is widely known to be available, *without* a referral, from a variety of centres. Tonti-Filippini proposes that the law should be carefully amended to 'balance the right to conscientiously object against the needs of a patient to know the availability of lawful services, and for the exercise of the right not to be overly disruptive in the provision of lawful services' (2013: 160). He believes, however, that the law should only require an objecting practitioner to inform the woman that other practitioners may be prepared to provide the service that she has requested.

Rights and responsibilities

Several ethicists describe sets of criteria for deciding whether a healthcare professional's claim to conscientious objection is ethically justified (Brock, 2008; Magelssen, 2012; Sulmasy, 2008; Wicclair, 2000). Magelssen (2012: 19) provides a particularly detailed evaluative framework, which states that conscientious objection ought to be accepted when:

1 Providing health care would seriously damage the healthcare professional's moral integrity by
    a constituting a serious violation . . .
    b . . . of a deeply held conviction
2 The objection has a plausible moral or religious rationale
3 The treatment is not considered an essential part of the healthcare professional's work
4 The burdens to the patient are acceptably small
    a The patient's condition is not life-threatening
    b Refusal does not lead to the patient not getting the treatment, or to unacceptable delay or expenses
    c Measures have been taken to reduce the burdens to the patient
5 The burdens to colleagues and healthcare institutions are acceptably small.

In addition, the claim to conscientious objection is strengthened if:

6 The objection is founded in medicine's own values
7 The medical procedure is new or of uncertain moral status.

Some healthcare professional codes of ethics and related position statements also specify, in detail, conditions and responsibilities of healthcare professionals who conscientiously refuse to provide a particular medical service (e.g see, Australian Nursing Federation, 2011; Australian Medical Association, 2013). These recognise that any exercise of a 'right' to conscientious objection also involves a series of duties. Healthcare professionals, in particular, have a duty to 'do no harm' to their patients.

On this basis, in order to minimise treatment delays or expense, objecting practitioners should communicate their objection to the patient at the earliest possible stage, preferably before a request for the objectionable treatment is made – perhaps via a notice in a waiting room, a brochure for new patients or an announcement on a website. As with any professional encounter, communicating an objection should be done with courtesy, sensitivity and respect. While the moral acceptability of referral will vary among healthcare professionals, where delay in treatment would be injurious, the objector should at least ensure that the patient is informed about the nature and alternative availability of the requested treatment (Magelssen, 2012).

Employed staff also have a responsibility to inform their supervisors of any relevant deeply held moral values and potential conflicts of conscience within their workplace setting so that, wherever possible, potential conflicts of conscience can be avoided or accommodated. There may, however, be reasonable limits to these claims of conscience. For instance, although most professional codes of practice and laws allow nurses to conscientiously object to direct assistance in abortion and sterilisation procedures, they may not be justified in refusing pre- or post-operative care for patients undergoing these procedures (outside of direct preparation for surgery), or for providing care in ways that express their moral disapproval of the patient's choices (Dickens & Cook, 2000: 74). It is also generally accepted that a healthcare professional's duty to provide potentially life-saving treatment overrides any claim to conscientious objection (Dickens & Cook, 2000; Magelssen, 2012; Sulmasy, 2008). In many jurisdictions, this is mandated by law.

Conclusion

In view of the ethical character of healthcare, and its role as the guardian of personal moral integrity, conscience is indeed the 'friend' of the healthcare professional. Conscience enables us to choose and act in accordance with our deepest and most personal moral convictions and aspirations. It follows that an important consequence of conscientious healthcare practice is that healthcare professionals will sometimes refuse to either deliver or refer for medical services that conflict with their deeply held moral convictions. Conscientious objection need not, however, be undertaken in a discriminatory or intolerant manner, or exercised in such a way that patient health is compromised or access to requested services is deliberately impeded. Conscientious objection can have a legitimate place in contemporary healthcare, so long as it is focused upon morally objectionable services (not patients), and exercised with responsibility and courtesy towards others. For the most part, rather than *restricting* services, the promotion and protection of conscientious practice serves to enhance the *delivery* of healthcare that is marked by practical wisdom, compassion and justice. In this regard, conscience is the 'friend', not only of healthcare professionals, but also the community in which they practise, and is worthy of respect, accommodation and protection.

Reflective exercises

11.1 In this chapter, it is proposed that conscience is 'an intellectual activity that arises in particular ethical deliberations'.

- Summarise in your own words the definition of conscience presented in this chapter.
- What are some of the social, cultural, experiential, clinical and spiritual influences that may have shaped your own moral conscience?
- Reflecting on your own clinical practice, have there been any situations where you have appealed to your conscience to assist in decision-making processes?

11.2 What may be some of the benefits of and limitations to freedom of conscience for healthcare professionals in the provision of clinical care? Who may these benefits and limitations be most directed towards?

11.3 The chapter explores the notion of 'moral distress' with connection to restrictions placed upon freedom of conscience.

- What are some of the physical and mental symptoms consistent with moral distress as described in evidence-based literature?

- Reflecting on your own clinical practice, have there been any conflicting ethical situations where you may have experienced moral distress? What were your effective (or non-effective) methods for addressing this conflict?
- What clinical-based policies and procedures, or professional codes, position statements or support systems, are available to you in responding to an experience of moral distress in practice?

11.4 Define what is meant by the term 'conscientious objection'.

- What are some of the key elements presented by Magelssen cited in this chapter that constitute an authentic claim of conscientious objection in the provision of care?
- Identify what would be an example of a discriminatory action by the healthcare professional in refusing to participate in the provision of treatment to a patient.
- Could a connection be made between a healthcare professional conscientiously objecting to their direct participation in a treatment or procedure that violates their reasoned moral conscience and patient advocacy? Explore this question in the provision of healthcare to vulnerable members of the community, such as the disabled, cognitively impaired or members of culturally and linguistically diverse groups.
- Review the section '"Objections" to conscientious objection'. Identify the key arguments in terms of human rights and principlism that would oppose a healthcare professional's ability to conscientiously object in clinical practice.

References

Australian Medical Association (2013). *Conscientious Objection.*

Australian Medical Council (2009). Good Medical Practice: A Code of Conduct for Doctors in Australia.

Australian Nursing Federation (2011). *Conscientious Objection.*

Birchley, G. (2011). A clear case for conscience in healthcare practice. *Journal of Medical Ethics*, 38: 13–17.

Blustein, J. & Fleischman, A. R. (1995). The pro-life maternal-fetal medicine physician: a problem of integrity. *The Hastings Center Report*, 22(5): 22–6.

Brock, D. W. (2008). Conscientious refusal by physicians and pharmacists: who is obligated to do what, and why? *Theoretical Medical Bioethics* 29: 187–200.

Cantor, J. D. (2009). Conscientious objection gone awry: Restoring selfless professionalism in medicine. *New England Journal of Medicine*, 360(15): 1484–5.

Cantor, J. & Baum, K. (2004). The limits of conscientious objection: May pharmacists refuse to fill prescriptions for emergency contraception? *New England Journal of Medicine*, 351(19): 2008–12.

Charo, R. A. (2005). The celestial fire of conscience: Refusing to deliver medical care. *New England Journal of Medicine*, 352: 2471–3

Corley, M. C. (2002). Nurse moral distress: A proposed theory and research agenda. *Nursing Ethics*, 9(6): 636–50.

Curlin, F. A., Lawrence, R. E., Chin, M. H. & Lantos, J. D. (2007). Religion, conscience and controversial clinical practices. *New England Journal of Medicine*, 356(6): 593–600.

Davis, S., Schrader, V. & Belcheir, M. J. (2012). Influencers of ethical beliefs and the impact on moral distress and conscientious objection. *Nursing Ethics*, 19(738): 738–49.

Dickens, B. (2009). Legal protection and limits of conscientious objection: When conscientious objection is unethical. *Medicine and Law*, 28: 337–47.

Dickens, B. M. & Cook, R. J. (2000). The scope and limits of conscientious objection. *International Journal of Gynecology & Obstetrics*, 71: 71–7.

—— (2011). Conscientious commitment to women's health. *International Journal of Gynecology and Obstetrics*, 113: 163–6.

Epstein, E. G. & Delgado, S. (2010). Understanding and addressing moral distress. *The Online Journal of Issues in Nursing*, 15(3): Manuscript 1.

Fisher, A. (2012). *Catholic bioethics for a new millennium*. New York: Cambridge University Press.

Gallagher, A. (2010). Moral distress and moral courage in everyday nursing practice. *The Online Journal of Issues in Nursing*, 16(2): 1–8.

Gregory, D. (2009). Catholic, a chemist but he won't sell the pill. *The Sydney Morning Herald*, 11 October. Retrieved 20 February 2014 from <http://www.smh.com.au/national/catholic-a-chemist-but-he-wont-sell-the-pill-20091010-grka.html>.

Harris, L. H. (2012). Recognizing conscience in abortion provision. *New England Journal of Medicine*, 367(11): 981–3.

Johnstone, M. (2009). *Bioethics: A nursing perspective* (5th ed.). Sydney: Churchill Livingstone/Elsevier.

Kaczor, C. (2012). Conscientious objection and health care: A reply to Bernard Dickens. *Christian Bioethics*, 18(1): 59–71.

Laabs, C. A. (2009). Nurses and conundrums of conscience. *Forum on Public Policy: A Journal of the Oxford Round Table*, 1: 1–19.

Lawrence, R. E. & Curlin, F. A. (2007). Clash of definitions: Controversies about conscience in medicine. *American Journal of Bioethics*, 7(12): 10–14.

Magelssen, M. (2012). When should conscientious objection be accepted? *Journal of Medical Ethics*, 38: 18–21.

Mayoh, L. (2009). God before contraception. *The Sunday Telegraph*, 10 October. Retrieved 20 February 2014 from <http://www.dailytelegraph.com.au/god-before-contraception/story-e6freuy9-1225785346498>.

Morton, N. T. & Kirkwood, K. W. (2009). Conscience and conscientious objection of health-care professionals refocusing the issue. *HEC Forum* 21(4): 351–64.

Murphy, S. & Genuis, S. J. (2013). Freedom of conscience in health care: Distinctions and limits. *Journal of Bioethical Inquiry*, 10: 347–54.

Murray, J. S. (2010). Moral courage in healthcare: Acting ethically even in the presence of risk. *The Online Journal of Issues in Nursing*, 15(3): Manuscript 2.

Nursing and Midwifery Board of Australia (2008). *A Code of Ethics for Nurses in Australia*.

O'Rourke, A., De Crespigny, L. & Pyman, A. (2013). Abortion and conscientious objection: The new battleground. *Monash University Law Review*, 38(3): 87–119.

Pellegrino. E. D. (2002). The physician's conscience, conscience clauses, and religious belief: A Catholic perspective. *Fordham Urban Law Journal*, 30(1): 221–44.

Pharmacy Board of Australia (2010). *Pharmacy Code of Conduct for Registered Health Practitioners*.

Rolfe, P. (2013). Melbourne doctor's abortion stance may be punished. *Herald Sun*, 28 April. Retrieved 20 February 2014 from <http://www.theaustralian.com.au/news/melbourne-doctors-abortion-stance-may-be-punished/story-e6frg6n6-1226631128438>.

Savulescu J. (2006). Conscientious objection in medicine. *British Medical Journal*, 332: 294–7.

Smith, P. (2013). Abortion debate: the right to refuse referral. *Australian Doctor*, 7 November. Retrieved 20 February 2014 from <http://www.australiandoctor.com.au/news/news-insight/abortion-debate-the-right-to-refuse-referral>.

Strickland, S. (2012). Conscientious objection in medical students: A questionnaire survey. *Journal of Medical Ethics*, 38: 22–5.

Sulmasy, D. (2008). What is conscience and why is respect for it so important? *Theoretical Medical Bioethics*, 29(3): 135–49.

Tonti-Filippini, N. (2013). *About bioethics*. Ballarat: Connor Court.

United Nations (1966). *International Covenant on Civil and Political Rights (ICCPR)*. Retrieved 20 February 2014 from <http://www.ohcr.org/en/professionalinterest/pages/ccpr.aspx>.

Wicclair, M. R. (2000). Conscientious objection in medicine. *Bioethics*, 14: 205–27.

—— (2008). Is conscientious objection incompatible with a physician's professional obligations? *Theoretical Medical Bioethics*, 29: 171–85.

12 Is there a right to life and a right to die?

Frank Brennan

The legal and moral dimensions of rights talk

The person who asks, 'Is there a right to life or a right to die?' may be looking for a legal answer or a moral one. The inquirer looking for a legal answer may be wanting to know what are their present legal entitlements or obligations: 'What must I do to avoid trouble with the law?' or 'What can I avoid doing without running into trouble with the law?' For example, the nurse may want to know whether she has a duty to assist with an abortion or the duty to assist a patient to commit suicide. The patient may want to know whether they can terminate a pregnancy without fear of criminal sanction or involve their spouse in assisting with their death, confident that their partner will not face prosecution after the peaceful death which would come more quickly than if the patient simply accepted good palliative care. The questioner looking for a moral answer is not so much interested in the present way of dealing with life at either end of the life-cycle, but rather with pondering how best we and our society might in future deal with people in such situations. The moral questioner is concerned with asking, 'What ought we do? In a more ideal world, what ought we do? Even in a messy and broken world, what ought we do? How could laws and policies best be formulated to regulate, guide and determine how people respond and act when confronting life at either end of the life-cycle?' When speaking of the right to die, we are usually wrestling with the moral dilemma of how best to order the doctor–patient relationship, how best to provide legal underpinning for the decisions made by patients and their next of kin, and how best to allow a patient to decide their options for life or death. If there is a right to die, it is a right to die at the time and in the manner of one's choosing?

It may be that 'rights talk' can help. However, some might find 'rights talk' a distraction. They might find it more useful to speak of values such as autonomy and dignity, which need to be respected and upheld in all decision-making. Even when rights talk is helpful, it is not usually as easy as invoking rights as trumps. Asserting a right does not necessarily settle the matter; there are limits to rights. My right to free speech is limited by my neighbour's right to a good reputation. My right to private property is limited by the public interest or common good requiring that land be available for resumption by a public authority wanting the land for a public purpose – although, of course, only after due process and payment of just compensation. Some talk of rights would more accurately be discussion about liberties. In March 2014, the Australian Attorney-General spoke of 'the right to be a bigot' (George Brandis, cited in Wilson, 2014). There is a right to free speech. However, that right might be abused, and it often is. One abuse of the right is the making of bigoted or hateful remarks. The making of such remarks is not the exercise of a right; it is merely the exercise of a liberty. I do not have the duty to allow the bigot to speak their mind in the public square. I have the liberty to drown them out. I have the duty to allow the free speech of someone who is not speaking in a defamatory, bigoted or hateful way, and who is not interfering with the rights of others.

In most societies, the law will stay in step with the community's moral sense about right and wrong, about the big issues like life and death. The law will sometimes be a little ahead or more often lagging a little behind. When the law is out of step with popular sentiment – especially the more primitive expression of that sentiment in opinion polls – it will often be because the law has to take account of a range of circumstances and possibilities. The law might then turn a blind eye to some breaches, in part because breaches at the edges are always envisaged and breaches might still be consistent with the spirit of the law. A change in the law would require a change to the contours that human relations or human actions usually follow. The simplest example is a legal speed limit on the roads. When the limit is set at 100 km/h, the driver has the right to drive safely at any speed up to 100 km/h. The police will allow a margin of error or just a margin of wilful latitude. Some drivers will always drive 5 km/h over the speed limit when they consider it safe to do so. There is no point increasing the speed limit to 105 km/h, as the same drivers will now drive at 110 km/h.

The law might continue to stipulate that doctors do no harm, allowing them to administer sedatives to palliate pain even though this might incidentally shorten the life of the patient. Some doctors will administer excessive sedatives, intending that this will more quickly shorten the life of the patient. They will not be prosecuted. Were the law to be changed to accommodate this practice, it is then more likely that the lethal injection would be used routinely. A change to the law would render the contours for decision-making more porous. While the law prohibits the administration of the lethal injection, there is still plenty of discernment and scope for disagreement among family members deciding how much sedation to authorise for the dying loved one. Were the law to permit the lethal injection, there would be even greater scope for bitter family disagreement about whether the loved one should now live or die, and the matter would not be concluded to everyone's satisfaction just because the dying person had earlier given a directive before being less able to communicate or to reason. Some family members professing to know the dying one's real personality best might be worried that the directive could well have been reversed.

Belgium – one of the few jurisdictions to have legalised euthanasia – provides an indicator of where the rights discussion may be headed once the principle of 'do no harm' is abandoned. This is one of the realms of human activity where a 'slippery slope' is evident. The Belgian Society of Intensive Care Medicine (2014) recently issued a statement on end-of-life issues, expressing the belief that 'shortening the dying process by administering sedatives beyond what is needed for patient comfort can be not only acceptable but in many cases desirable'. The society's first statement of principle is:

> Suffering should be avoided at all times. When the intensive care team reaches a consensus that current treatment no longer has any meaningful perspective and/or is disproportionate and/or is in conflict with advance directives, then it is ethically justified – and even appropriate – to stop this treatment.

The society lists a number of complementary principles, including:

> There is no clear ethical distinction between withholding/withdrawing supportive therapy and increasing doses of sedative/opioid substances in patients in whom further treatment is no longer considered beneficial.

It is stated that 'it must be made clear that the final decision is made by the care team and not by the relatives'.

The late American physician-ethicist Ed Pellegrino (2001) once pointed out:

> The slippery slope is not a myth. Historically it has been a reality in world affairs. Once a moral precept is breached a psychological and logical process

is set in motion which follows what I would call the law of infinite regress of moral exceptions. One exception leads logically and psychologically to another. In small increments a moral norm eventually obliterates itself. The process always begins with some putative good reason, like compassion, freedom of choice, or liberty. By small increments it overwhelms its own justifications.

When considering the right to life and the right to die, we are usually concerned with issues such as abortion, euthanasia, physician-assisted suicide, medically assisted dying and palliative sedation. In this chapter, I will focus on end-of-life issues, rather than beginning-of-life ones, simply because the beginning-of-life issues are basically static, legally and morally, in societies like the United Kingdom, the United States, Canada and Australia. The moral divide is clearly drawn between those who espouse the right to life of the foetus before birth, and especially after viability, and those who espouse the mother's right to choose up until birth, even after viability. The former espouse the right to life for all persons, including the unborn; the latter do not invoke a right to life for a person until birth; there are even some of them who would not invoke the right to life until some time after birth, when the baby satisfies their added criteria for personhood. Even if the law accords a mother a right to choose life or death for her child up until the moment of birth, there is a need to concede that the duty to assist the mother to abort her child ought not be imposed on the nurse or doctor who has a conscientious objection to abortion.

Diverse philosophical views

In contemporary discourse, there is often a meshing of legal and moral concepts by speaking about rights as 'human rights'. When discussing what ought be recognised as a human right, we inevitably need to fall back on our primary philosophical approach to determining what is right and wrong – what is a necessary precondition for human flourishing and for justice. The utilitarian will argue that something is right because it provides the greatest benefit to the greatest number (or some variant on that calculus). Proponents of natural law, such as legal scholar and philosopher John Finnis, advocate that something is a precondition for the structuring of society and relations, enhancing the prospect that all persons might achieve their full human flourishing as members of that society and while engaged in those relationships. The Kantian, forever seeking universal rules or maxims in the footsteps of Immanuel Kant (2012), will propose that this entitlement for all and that duty imposed on all will result in all persons acting 'in such a way that you treat humanity, whether in your own person or in the person of any other, never merely as a means, but always at the same time as an end'. The Rawlsian, following the path of the contract theorists culminating in the writings of John Rawls, will imagine themselves behind a veil of ignorance, not knowing what their lot in life will be, agreeing on the preconditions for all persons wanting to live in society harmoniously. The Rawlsian draws up a list of basic liberties to be enjoyed by all, and a set of rules for distributing the unequal things in life – including public offices – so as to maximise benefits for all, especially the least advantaged.

Once we investigate much of the contemporary discussion about human rights, we find that often the intended recipients of rights do not include all human beings, but only those with certain capacities or those who share sufficient common attributes with the decision-makers. It is always at the edges that there is real work for human rights discourse to do. Speaking at the London School of Economics on 'Religious Faith and Human Rights', Rowan Williams (2008), when Archbishop of Canterbury, boldly and correctly asserted:

> The question of foundations for the discourse of non-negotiable rights is not one that lends itself to simple resolution in secular terms; so it is not at all odd if diverse ways of framing this question in religious terms flourish so persistently. The uncomfortable truth is that a purely secular account of human rights is always going to be problematic if it attempts to establish a language of rights as a supreme and non-contestable governing concept in ethics.

No one should pretend that the discourse about universal ethics and inalienable rights has a firmer foundation than it actually has. Once we abandon any religious sense that the human person is created in the image and likeness of God, and that God has commissioned even the powerful to act justly, love tenderly and walk humbly, it may be difficult to maintain a human rights commitment to the weakest and most vulnerable in society. It may come down to the vote, moral sentiment or tribal affiliations. And that will not be enough to extend human rights universally – especially at the beginning and end of life. In the name of utility, the society might not feel so impeded in limiting social inclusion to those like us – 'us' being the decision-makers who determine which common characteristics render embodied persons eligible for human rights protection. Nicholas Wolterstorff (2008) says, 'Our moral subculture of rights is as frail as it is remarkable. If the secularisation thesis proves true, we must expect that that subculture will have been a brief shining episode in the odyssey of human beings on earth.'

The concept of human rights has real work to do whenever those with power justify their solutions to social ills or political conflicts only on the basis of majority support, or by claiming the solutions will lead to an improved situation for the mainstream majority. Even if a particular solution is popular or maximises gains for the greatest number of people, it might still be wrong and objectionable. There is a need to have regard to the well-being of all members of the community. By invoking human rights, we affirm that every person's well-being needs to be considered by the state in ordering the common life of the community.

'Human rights' is the contemporary language for embracing, and the modern means of achieving, respect and dignity for all. Especially when considering rights and duties at the end of the life-cycle, we need to keep an eye on the effects of any laws or practices that are likely to impact on the vulnerable, including those with increasingly impaired cognitive capacity, and the marginalised of society, including those who do not have the financial resources to afford ongoing healthcare or the network of friendship, family and professional support to assist with making life-determining decisions.

Conceding that there are diverse strands of philosophical thought about right and wrong, rights and duties, most of us are prepared to leave the turf war to professional philosophers, satisfied that we have an intuitive sense about right and wrong that can be more finely honed by our being occasionally exposed to the different philosophical lines of inquiry. We have the benefit that, since World War II, the governments of nations have worked closely together to formulate various statements of human rights, drawn with assistance from philosophers of all strands and agreed to by actors from every culture and religious tradition on earth.

Rights in United Nations instruments

The United Nations' (UN) founding document on human rights, the Universal Declaration of Human Rights (UDHR), lists a set of human rights including: 'Everyone has the right to life, liberty and security of person.' It is a mistake just to list the rights set down in UN documents as if they were trump cards. They are not rights without limit. The UDHR concedes that limitations can be placed on the listed rights. Article 29(2) provides:

> In the exercise of his rights and freedoms, everyone shall be subject only to such limitations as are determined by law solely for the purpose of securing due recognition and respect for the rights and freedoms of others and of meeting the just requirements of morality, public order and the general welfare in a democratic society.

Once the UN was established, the nation-states engaged in the painstaking work of drawing up the two key covenants on rights, the International Covenant on Civil and Political Rights (ICCPR) and the International Covenant on Economic, Social and Cultural Rights (ICESCR). Many countries, having ratified these covenants, have also voluntarily signed additional protocols that require their governments to make regular reports to UN bodies setting out their compliance with these instruments. Thus the language of these instruments is not just idealistic; it is supported by agreements that make the language more normative, providing identifiable contours for the making and implementation of domestic legislation and policies.

Though conceding that governments can derogate from many of the enumerated rights during times of national emergency, these instruments single out some rights that can never be derogated. Included in the list of non-derogable rights is Article 6 of the ICCPR: 'Every human being has the inherent right to life. This right shall be protected by law. No one shall be arbitrarily deprived of his life.' Also included in the non-derogable list is Article 7, which provides that 'no one shall be subjected without his free consent to medical or scientific experimentation'.

Article 12 of the ICESCR provides that, 'The States Parties to the present Covenant recognise the right of everyone to the enjoyment of the highest attainable standard of physical and mental health.' However, all rights in the ICESCR – as distinct from the ICCPR –are subject to one further caveat: governments commit themselves with 'a view to achieving progressively the full realisation' of economic and social rights. It is conceded that the realisation of such rights requires significant government expenditure, which may not be available at present.

Some of the language of UN conventions is simply hortatory and idealistic, and some of it belongs to the idealism and morality of an earlier age. For example, the preamble of the Convention on the Rights of the Child harks back to the original Declaration of the Rights of the Child, which stipulates that 'the child, by reason of his physical and mental immaturity, needs special safe-guards and care, including appropriate legal protection, before as well as after birth'. Nowadays there is no UN commitment to protecting the unborn child from the decision of a mother who chooses to abort. Some UN language on rights is grossly inflated. For example, the preamble of the Constitution of the World Health Organization (2006) states: 'The enjoyment of the highest attainable standard of health is one of the fundamental rights of every human being without distinction of race, religion, political belief, economic or social condition.' These UN instruments are useful indicators of what constitutes common ground in the pursuit of justice and truth across cultures, religious faiths and national boundaries. The development of these instruments, as well as those of smaller collections of states, has placed rights talk central to the quest for the statement of ideals to be achieved by national laws and policies.

The constitutional protection of rights in domestic law

Democracies committed to the rule of law take two approaches to the domestic protection of rights at law. An increasing number of nation-states have a constitutional bill of rights or a human rights statute, which prevails over and assists in the interpretation of ordinary laws enacted by their parliaments. These legal instruments often contain broad terms requiring due process and equal protection of the laws for all citizens, and declaring open-ended rights without articulating corresponding duties, obligations or responsibilities. As new bioethical and medical ethical questions arise, disaffected citizens are able to challenge existing laws or government policies in the courts, thereby forcing the state to consider legal reform more quickly than might occur if there were to be reliance only on popular discontent being expressed at the ballot box or on the floor of the parliament. Canada and the United States are the exemplars of this first set of countries.

In the past, suicide was a criminal offence in most jurisdictions – not that one could ever prosecute an offender, because they would be dead. Rather, this made attempted suicide an offence. Though persons who attempted suicide unsuccessfully were rarely prosecuted, this law was thought to act as a deterrent to suicide, thereby buttressing the fundamental values of a society that espoused the dignity and worth of all human life. Once suicide was decrimin-alised, the question arose of whether it would be an offence to assist with a suicide. Most jurisdictions retained this offence, once again to underpin society's commitment to human life.

Section 7 of the Canadian Charter of Rights and Freedoms provides that:

> Everyone has the right to life, liberty and security of the person and the right not to be deprived thereof except in accordance with the principles of fundamental justice.

In *Rodriguez v British Columbia* (1993), the Supreme Court of Canada was asked to rule on the application of section 7 when it came to a person wanting physician-assisted suicide at the hands of a physician who was willing to assist. The argument was that the continuing law criminalising assistance with suicide was inconsistent with section 7, at least in those instances when the assistant was to be a competent physician enlisted with the informed consent of a mentally competent patient. Justice Sopinka wrote (1993: 606–7):

> The distinction between withdrawing treatment upon a patient's request ... and assisted suicide ... has been criticized as resting on a legal fiction ... However, the distinction drawn here is one based on intention – in the case of palliative care the intention is to ease pain, which has the effect of hastening death, while in the case of assisted suicide, the intention is undeniably to cause death.

Justice Sopinka concluded (1993: 608) that, 'To the extent that there is a consensus, it is that human life must be respected and we must be careful not to undermine the institutions that protect it.' Recently, the courts in British Columbia have had to consider cases in which the plaintiffs with incurable illnesses have argued that section 7 of the charter would support their claim of a right to assisted suicide. They start with the proposition that any person is entitled to commit suicide – that they have a right to commit suicide. With an illness that causes increasing physical incapacity, they argue they will be unable to commit suicide later in their illness unaided, and thus they would need to commit suicide earlier than they would need to were they to have the option of lawful assistance with suicide when they felt ready to die. By having to opt for suicide earlier, they argue that they are being deprived of life and that this is not 'in accordance with the principles of fundamental justice', and therefore that the prohibition of assisted suicide is unconstitutional, which means they have an entitlement to assistance with suicide at a time of their choosing, and the right to choose their time and method of death.

In the British Columbia Supreme Court, the plaintiffs – one of them suffering from amyotrophic lateral sclerosis (ALS) – won at first instance (*Carter v Canada*,

2012) but lost two to one on appeal (*Carter v Canada*, 2013). The Supreme Court of Canada, with its rights jurisprudence, will determine – regardless of the views of parliament – whether the prohibition on assisted suicide is unconstitutional, thereby deciding whether persons unable to effect suicide for themselves have a right to assistance – presumably from a medical practitioner. In the British Columbia Court of Appeal, two of the judges observed:

> [T]he societal consequences of permitting physician-assisted suicide in Canada – and indeed enshrining it as a constitutional right – are a matter of serious concern to many Canadians, and as is shown by the evidence reviewed by the trial judge in this case, no consensus on the subject is apparent, even among ethicists or medical practitioners (2013, Newbury and Saunders JJ).

But it will fall to the Supreme Court of Canada to make a decision. High-level, abstract statements such as the right to life being limitable only 'in accordance with the principles of fundamental justice' open the way for the courts to determine rights that parliament had never previously considered, and that courts had previously considered only on an incremental basis, deciding each case according to the common law.

Similarly in the United States, plaintiffs unable to help themselves to death will continue to petition the courts, arguing that other citizens have the right to commit suicide while they have an inhibited capacity to do so. Their argument will be that their request for assistance in committing suicide should not be refused by the law because such refusal amounts to a failure to accord due process or to provide equal protection of the laws of the United States. They argue that everyone should have access to death, regardless of their personal capacity to effect it. The issue, then, will be the limiting of the right to assisted suicide to those who are terminally ill, or to those who are terminally ill and enduring unbearable pain, or to those who are terminally ill, enduring unbearable pain, mentally competent and not depressed. To date, the US Supreme Court has held firm in denying a constitutional right to physician-assisted suicide, no matter what the sub-class of possible rights-holders. The two key cases, *Vacco v Quill* and *Washington v Glucksberg* were decided in 1997. A philosophers' brief from some of the world's leading political philosophers in the 1997 litigation argued:

> Just as it would be intolerable for government to dictate that doctors never be permitted to try to keep someone alive as long as possible, when that is what the patient wishes, so it is intolerable for government to dictate that doctors may never, under any circumstances, help someone to die who believes that further life means only degradation. (Dworkin & Zimroth, 1999: 44)

They went on to argue:

> From the patient's point of view, there is no morally pertinent difference
> between a doctor's terminating treatment that keeps him alive, if that is
> what he wishes, and a doctor's helping him to end his own life by providing
> lethal pills he may take himself, when ready, if that is what he wishes – except
> that the latter may be quicker and more humane ... If it is permissible for a
> doctor deliberately to withdraw medical treatment in order to allow death to
> result from a natural process, then it is equally permissible for him to help his
> patient hasten his own death more actively, if that is the patient's express
> wish. (1999: 44)

The philosophers' brief did not find favour with the Supreme Court – indeed,
the judges did not even quote it. They upheld state restrictions on assisted
suicide and other euthanasia practices while leaving the matter for further
agitation in the state legislatures and in the public forum. In *Vacco*, the court
unanimously and simply stated its view (1997: 801–2):

> We think the distinction between assisting suicide and withdrawing life
> sustaining treatment, a distinction widely recognised and endorsed in the
> medical profession and in our legal traditions, is both important and logical;
> it is certainly rational.

Concluding the brief judgment for the court, Chief Justice Rehnquist said:

> By permitting everyone to refuse unwanted medical treatment while prohib-
> iting anyone from assisting a suicide, New York law follows a longstanding
> and rational distinction.

He listed New York's reasons for recognising and acting on this distinction
(1997: 808–9):

> prohibiting intentional killing and preserving life; preventing suicide;
> maintaining physicians' role as their patients' healers; protecting vulnerable
> people from indifference, prejudice, and psychological and financial pressure
> to end their lives; and avoiding a possible slide towards euthanasia.

The court was left in no doubt that these were valid and important public
interests, which easily satisfied the constitutional requirement that a legislative
classification should bear a rational relation to some legitimate end, thereby
limiting any right to assistance when choosing the time and manner of one's
death.

In *Glucksberg* (1997), the court decided that an equivalent law prohibiting
assisted suicide did not violate the due process clause. Conceding that attitudes

to suicide had changed over time, Chief Justice Rehnquist said (1997: 719): 'Despite changes in medical technology and notwithstanding an increased emphasis on the importance of end-of-life decision making, we have not retreated from this prohibition.' Wanting to avoid a repetition of the Supreme Court's having become an arbiter on abortion regulations, the Chief Justice warned (1997: 720) of the dangers of the court expanding the concept of due process as 'guideposts for responsible decision making in this uncharted area are scarce and open-ended'. The court in 1997 was well aware that the issue of physician-assisted suicide was not going away any time soon, and that it was not to be finally resolved by the Supreme Court ruling for or against the right to physician administered death. The Chief Justice observed (1997: 735):

> Throughout the Nation, Americans are engaged in an earnest and profound debate about the morality, legality, and practicality of physician-assisted suicide. Our holding permits this debate to continue, as it should in a democratic society.

Justice O'Connor, with the support of Justices Ginsburg and Breyer, pointed out (1997: 737) that, although there was no constitutional right to commit suicide or to be assisted in suicide, there was no legal barrier to terminal patients in great pain 'obtaining medication, from qualified physicians, to alleviate that suffering, even to the point of causing unconsciousness and hastening death'. Even in the United States, the home of constitutional rights, it is not primarily a matter of delimiting a right to die, but rather of striking the appropriate balance between the interests of the autonomous, self-determining, rational, terminal patient and the state's interests in protecting the weak and vulnerable. O'Connor concluded (1997: 737) with this consolation offered to reformers:

> Every one of us at some point may be affected by our own or a family member's terminal illness. There is no reason to think the democratic process will not strike the proper balance between the interests of terminally ill, mentally competent individuals who would seek to end their suffering and the State's interests in protecting those who might seek to end life mistakenly or under pressure. As the Court recognises, States are presently undertaking extensive and serious evaluation of physician-assisted suicide and other related issues.

It is no answer to these moral quandaries simply to argue that the voluntary death with informed consent of a person who is not depressed does not cause direct harm to any other person. Even if that were so, a legal regime that permitted such liberty would also create risks and added burdens for others.

The one-dimensional liberal envisages the paradigm case as the free, self-determining individual who has the personal resources to make all key life decisions without any social assistance or support. Though the argument is more complex, others of us envisage the paradigm case of the individual who craves a sphere of personal autonomy and a penumbra of social support around that sphere within a society where fundamental values are espoused. John Roberts, the present Chief Justice of the United States, said in his first graduation address at Georgetown University that we need to be 'learned in those wise restraints that make us free'. Even in those jurisdictions with a constitutional bill of rights, rights are not trumps.

Non-constitutional protection of rights in domestic law

Jurisdictions without bills of rights do not provide potential plaintiffs with the same opportunity to agitate potential rights in the courts. They are left more dependent on elected politicians legislating in the parliaments. Judges are left to apply and develop the common law incrementally, and to interpret statutes consistent with fundamental human rights. But even in these jurisdictions, there is an acknowledgement of the right to autonomy and the right to bodily integrity. The self-determining patient has the right to refuse treatment. The patient has a right to be free from pain. But that does not translate readily into a right to assisted suicide or a right to medically assisted dying.

The most notable cases in the media relate to patients who are not elderly, and who are in the final stages of a terminal illness. They tend to be young rugby players rendered quadriplegic, who want to end their lives rather than face decades in a wheelchair, or those like the 51-year-old Debbie Purdy in the United Kingdom, who has been confined to a wheelchair since 2001, having been diagnosed with multiple sclerosis in 1995. In October 2008, when first going to court to seek the order clarifying that the Director of Public Prosecutions would not prosecute her husband if he were to assist with her suicide once she could no longer control her bodily functions, she said:

> We are not asking for the law to be changed for it to be made compulsory for people at the end of their lives to be dragged off to the knacker's yard. But this should be one of the choices available and for it to be available we need to be clear on the law. (cited in Beckford, 2008)

Purdy (cited in Beckford, 2008) told the court:

> My dearest wish would be to die with dignity in my own home, with my husband and other loved ones around me ... My husband has said that he would assist me, and if necessary face a prison sentence, but I am not prepared to put him in this position for a number of reasons. I love him and do not want him to risk ending up in prison. As long as the DPP will not clarify his policy on prosecutions in these circumstances, I worry that as my husband is black and a foreigner, this makes him a more likely target for prosecution.

One could not but be moved by her plea. The United Kingdom Director of Public Prosecutions provided guidelines including:

> prosecution is less likely to be required if:
> - the victim had reached a voluntary, clear, settled and informed decision to commit suicide;
> - the suspect was wholly motivated by compassion;
> - the actions of the suspect, although sufficient to come within the definition of the offence, were of only minor encouragement or assistance;
> - the suspect had sought to dissuade the victim from taking the course of action which resulted in his or her suicide;
> - the actions of the suspect may be characterised as reluctant encouragement or assistance in the face of a determined wish on the part of the victim to commit suicide;
> - the suspect reported the victim's suicide to the police and fully assisted them in their enquiries into the circumstances of the suicide or the attempt and his or her part in providing encouragement or assistance.
>
> (Crown Prosecution Service, 2010)

Chances are that these guidelines would avoid prosecution of those few cases where palliative care is unable to control pain, and where the loss of autonomy of the patient occasions extraordinary angst and suffering. The formulation of prosecution guidelines does not have the same dramatic effect as the constitutional ruling on rights by the Supreme Court of Canada or the Supreme Court of the United States. But it has produced much the same result to date. It is not a matter of defining any right to die, but of delimiting the circumstances in which one is or is not likely to be prosecuted for assisting a loved one to die.

In those jurisdictions without a constitutional bill of rights, it is usually possible for the courts to resolve conflicts without the need for bold statements about rights. In 2009, Western Australian Chief Justice Wayne Martin gave a very sensible, uncontroversial decision in *Brightwater Care Group v Rossiter*

(2009). Mr Christian Rossiter was a profoundly disabled quadriplegic who was receiving nutrition and hydration through a percutaneous endoscopic gastro-stomy (PEG). He had had enough of life, and wanted his carers at Bridgewater Care to discontinue feeding him. Chief Justice Martin said (2009: 234):

> It is important I think to emphasise at the outset what this case is not about. It is not about euthanasia. Nor is it about physicians providing lethal treat-ments to patients who wish to die. Nor is it about the right to life or even the right to death.

The judge said that if Mr Rossiter, having received competent medical advice, decided to request Bridgewater to cease administering nutrition and hydration, then in the absence of any revocation of that direction by Rossiter, Bridgewater should cease to provide nutrition and hydration. There would be no risk of criminal liability. The only risk would arise if the caregiver were to continue feeding without consent and direction, because that could be an assault or a trespass on the person of Mr Rossiter.

This was nothing like the case of a person in a persistent vegetative state without the competence to decide and unable to communicate with the care-giver. As the judge made plain (2009: 237):

> Mr Rossiter is not a child, nor is he terminally ill, nor dying. He is not in a vegetative state, nor does he lack the capacity to communicate his wishes. There is therefore no question of other persons making decisions on his behalf.

Chief Justice Martin decided (2009: 241) that:

> Mr Rossiter has the right to determine whether or not he will continue to receive the services and treatment provided by Brightwater and, at common law, Brightwater would be acting unlawfully by continuing to provide treat-ment contrary to Mr Rossiter's wishes.

It is not only illegal, but also immoral, for a person to trespass without consent on the body of a competent person who specifically refuses consent to the trespass. It is not only against the law. It is wrong. It is morally objectionable. One should not trespass on the bodies of the mentally competent without consent.

Is there a right to die?

Euthanasia advocates speak with some ambivalence about the policy objectives of reformers in this field. Undertaking a review of the Exit International website will provide evidence to support such a claim. On the one hand, the group agitates for the right of any person to control their life and to take their life, regardless of their physical health or pain. It suggests that the state should not impede the provision or availability of substances like Nembutal so that citizens might always be assured a simple, dignified way of ending their lives, even if they are simply sick of living. Recently, Exit International founder and euthanasia advocate Dr Philip Nitschke gave the example of a couple who decided to consume Nembutal together because one did not want to go on living were the other to die of cancer (Brennan, 2014). On the other hand, euthanasia advocates concede that the only prospect of legislative change will be with the design of a law that contains stringent safeguards and preconditions. Presumably they think the safeguards can be removed or gradually loosened over time once we cross the medico-legal Rubicon of 'Do not intentionally kill' (Brennan, 2014).

Euthanasia advocates focus principally on the needs of those autonomous, resourceful persons wanting to end their lives. They point out that Nembutal is better than hanging – not just for the deceased, but also for those left behind. Concerns about others feeling pressured by relatives to consider death as an option are discounted (Brennan, 2014). The concerns of persons with disabilities are also discounted. The 2011 ComRes Poll (2011) in the United Kingdom should give us pause before extending further the liberty of medical practitioners wanting to facilitate death. ComRes asked 553 disabled persons:

> If there were a change in the law on assisted suicide would you be concerned about any of the following?'
> - Pressure being placed on you to end your life prematurely
>   Yes: 35%
>   No: 51%
>   Don't know: 12%
> - Pressure being placed on other disabled people to end their lives prematurely
>   Yes: 70%
>   No: 15%
>   Don't know: 12%
> - It being detrimental to the way that disabled people are viewed by society as a whole
>   Yes: 56%

Those who support the legalisation of euthanasia usually proceed by quoting cases of mentally competent, consenting patients who are not depressed but who are suffering unbearable pain, and are facing terminal illness. The easiest and most compelling case to consider is the patient whose relatives fully support the proposed euthanasia. There is no suggestion that the relatives are exerting undue influence on the patient for their own self-interested reasons. There are good palliative care facilities available, so it is not as if the patient is under duress, feeling that they have no option but death. The patient has a good and trusting relationship with their medical team. Under existing law and policy, there is every prospect that such a patient will be given increased doses of pain relief, which will hasten death. They might even be euthanised, with law enforcement agencies turning a blind eye or being oblivious to what has occurred, with the result of no legal action being taken.

Law professor and ethicist Margaret Somerville warns that we need to keep in mind an old saying in human rights: 'Nowhere are human rights more threatened than when we act purporting to do only good.' She writes (2014b: 224):

> When the good we seek is the relief of serious suffering, our moral intuition that it is wrong to intentionally kill another human being can be overwhelmed. Such intuitions are important guides in making good ethical decisions. And while we ignore our feelings at our ethical peril, our emotional reactions to an individual person's suffering need to become 'examined emotions' if we are to avoid the danger of their misleading us ethically.

Insofar as rights talk helps in resolving these moral conundrums, we can state that everyone has the right to life; deciding whether to commit suicide unassisted is a personal moral decision and is not prohibited by law; even if there were a right to die at the time and in the manner of one's choosing, that would not necessarily entail a duty on the state or on physicians to assist; and the state has a role in balancing the interests and protection of vulnerable people, in maintaining the integrity of the doctor–patient relationship and in upholding the value of life – that is, respect for the life of each person and respect for life in general in society. The right to die cannot be supported, but the right to be allowed to die can be. Its limits are marked by the enactment of laws and policies aimed at enhancing the autonomy and dignity of all persons. Depending on the constitutional arrangements in place, that balance will ultimately be struck by courts or parliaments. The contours and limits of choice will be somewhat porous, depending on the culture of the society and the trust placed in doctors. As Somerville (2014a) argues, we need to be passionately in favour of killing the pain while remaining adamantly opposed to killing the person with pain.

Reflective exercises

12.1 Review the Belgian Society of Intensive Care Medicine end-of-life statement and contrast it with Pellegrino's assertion that the 'slippery slope' argument in healthcare ethics is 'not a myth'. Is there any evidence in countries that have legalised assisted dying and/or euthanasia of a slippery slope effect occurring in end-of-life care?

12.2 List the different philosophical approaches to human rights discourse presented in this chapter. Apply these different approaches to end-of-life ethics. What are the similarities and main differences in these approaches? Do you see evidence of such philosophical approaches in your own clinical practice or in society?

12.3 This chapter presents the following statement by the former Archbishop of Canterbury, Rowan Williams: 'The uncomfortable truth is that a purely secular account of human rights is always going to be problematic if it attempts to establish a language of rights as a supreme and non-contestable governing concept in ethics.' Do you agree or disagree with this statement, and why?

12.4 Articulating a utilitarian perspective, this chapter states that, 'Even if a particular solution is popular or maximises gains for the greatest number of people, it might still be wrong and objectionable.' What are some of the complexities in legislating in favour of assisted dying and/or euthanasia and the protection of vulnerable members of society, or advocating for the common good at the end of life?

12.5 The chapter makes the following statement about human rights charters: 'It is a mistake just to list the rights set down in UN documents as if they were trump cards. They are not rights without limit.' What are some of the limitations in society that may impact on the codifying of various international human rights charters in contemporary law?

12.6 Review the various international human rights charters presented in this chapter. How may these charters provide support or defence against legalising of assisted dying and/or euthanasia in society?

12.7 The chapter makes the following statement: 'As new bioethical and medical ethical questions arise, disaffected citizens are able to challenge existing laws or government policies in the courts, thereby forcing the state to consider legal reform more quickly than might occur if there were to be reliance only on popular discontent being expressed at the ballot box or on the floor of the parliament.' Generally, democracies committed to the rule of law take two approaches to the domestic protection of rights at law. What are these two distinct approaches, and what connections can be made to human rights and ethical dilemmas for health professionals in provision of care at the end of life? Review the *Rossiter* case in this chapter to explore this discussion.

12.8   'The right to die cannot be supported, but the right to be allowed to die can be.' Do you agree or disagree with this statement? Why?

References

Beckford, M. (2008). Debbie Purdy demands Director of Public Prosecutions spell out law on assisted suicide. Retrieved 20 April 2014 from <http://www.telegraph.co.uk/news/uknews/3123290/Debbie-Purdy-demands-Director-of-Public-Prosecutions-spell-out-law-on-assisted-suicide.html>.

Belgian Society of Intensive Care Medicine (2014). 'Piece' of mind: End of life in the intensive care unit. Statement of the Belgian Society of Intensive Care Medicine. *Journal of Critical Care*, 29(1): 174–5.

Brennan, F. (2014). Discussing a good death with Philip Nitschke. *Eureka Street*, 24(3). Retrieved 20 August 2014 from <http://www.eurekastreet.com.au/article.aspx?aeid=38971#.VENBByhqPa4>.

ComRes (2011). Scope assisted suicide survey. Retrieved 25 April 2014 from <http://www.comres.co.uk/polls/DPP_Assisted_suicide_tables_March_2011.pdf>.

Crown Prosecution Service (2010). Policy for prosecutors in respect of cases of encouraging or assisting suicide. United Kingdom: Director of Public

Prosecutions. Retrieved 20 March 2014 from <http://www.cps.gov.uk/publications/prosecution/assisted_suicide_policy.html>.

Dworkin, R. & Zimroth, P. L. (1999). Brief of Ronald Dworkin, Thomas Nagel, Robert Nozick, John Rawls, Thomas Scanlon, and Judith Jarvis Thomson as *Amici Curiae* in support of respondents. *Issues in Law & Medicine*, 15(2): 183–98.

Kant, I. (2012) *Groundwork for the metaphysics of morals*, eds M. McGregor & J. Timmerman. Cambridge: Cambridge University Press.

Pellegrino, E. (2001) Physician-assisted suicide and euthanasia: Rebuttals of rebuttals. The moral prohibition remains. *Journal of Medicine and Philosophy*, 26(1): 93–100.

Somerville, M. (2014a). *Death talk* (2nd ed.). Montreal: McGill-Queens University Press.

—— (2014b). Exploring interactions between pain, suffering and the law. In N. J. Palpant & R. M. Green (eds). *Suffering and Bioethics*. Oxford: Oxford University Press, pp. 201–24.

UNICEF (1989). *Convention of the Rights of the Child*. Retrieved 20 February 2014 from <http://www.unicef.org/crc>.

United Nations (1948). *Universal Declaration of Human Rights*. Retrieved 20 February 2014 from <http://www.un.org/en/documents/udhr>.

—— (1966a). *International Covenant on Civil and Political Rights (ICCPR)*. Retrieved 20 February 2014 from <http://www.ohchr.org/en/professionalinterest/pages/ccpr.aspx>.

—— (1966b). *International Covenant on Economic Social and Cultural Rights (ICESCR)*. Retrieved 20 February 2014 from <http://www.ohchr.org/EN/ProfessionalInterest/Pages/CESCR.aspx>.

Williams, R. (2008). *Religious faith and human rights*. Retrieved 20 February 2014 from <http://www.lse.ac.uk/publicEvents/pdf/20080501_RowanWilliams.pdf>.

Wilson. L (2014). People have a right to be bigots, says Brandis. Retrieved 20 February 2014 from <http://www.theaustralian.com.au/national-affairs/people-have-a-right-to-be-bigots-says-brandis/story-fn59niix-1226863654303>.

Wolterstorff, N. (2008). *Justice: Rights and wrongs*. Princeton, NJ: Princeton University Press.

World Health Organization (2006). *Constitution of the World Health Organisation*. Retrieved 20 February 2014 from <http://www.who.int/governance/eb/who_constitution_en.pdf>.

Cases

Brightwater Care Group v Rossiter [2009] WASC 229.

Carter v Canada (Attorney General) 2012 BCSC 886.

Carter v Canada (Attorney General) (2013) 2013 BCCA 435.

Rodriguez v British Columbia [1993] 3 SCR 519.

Vacco v Quill 521 US 793 (1997).

Washington v Glucksberg 521 US 702 (1997).

13 When does human life begin? A theological, philosophical and scientific analysis

Norman Ford and Joanne Grainger

At the heart of many contemporary healthcare ethical debates is the question of when does human life begin. In February 2012, the prestigious *Journal of Medical Ethics* published an article titled 'After birth abortion: Why should the baby live?' by Australian ethicists Alberto Giubilini and Francesca Minerva (2012). This controversial article affirmed the authors' position that 'after-birth abortion' should be morally permissible in all cases where abortion is also permissible, including cases where the newborn is not disabled. Following its publication, the large portion of international responses to the article vehemently opposed the moral premises articulated by the authors that essentially supported infanticide. However, such a controversial premise is not new in historical or ethical discourse. Infanticide – the intentional killing of an infant by the mother – has been a part of many cultural practices over the centuries, from ancient Sparta to the more recent practice of intentionally killing newborn infants due to economic, cultural or social pressures placed on mothers and families. In 1988, Australian ethicists Helga Kuhse and Peter Singer also presented the argument that infanticide may be ethically justifiable in their book *Should the Baby Live? The Problem of Handicapped Infants*. A theological, philosophical and scientific analysis of the question of when human life begins can present some accord, but with contemporary ethical discourse from healthcare ethicists such as Kuhse and Singer (1988, 1990), Giubilini and Minerva (2012) and Julian Savulescu, there is an increasing divergence on what was once a universally accepted norm: that human life has moral inviolability from conception. This chapter will explore this issue by presenting some of the contemporary views, including theological, philosophical and scientific perspectives, as well as the cultural and historical influences on the question of when does human life begin. A particular focus to this discussion will be from a Christian anthropological framework, with an emphasis on the moral teachings of the Catholic Church.

Commencing this diverse discussion, the chapter will also start 'in the beginning' (Gen. 1:1). Human life as a divine gift from God has its origins in the Old Testament. The Book of Genesis projects a noble view of human dignity in its account of the creation of the first human beings, Adam and Eve. God said:

> Let us make man in our image, in the likeness of ourselves . . . God created man in the image of himself, in the image of God he created him, male and female he created them. (Gen. 1:26–7)

The life of a human is a unity of flesh and blood, heart, soul and experiences. One may be poor, infirm or lowly, but the value of human life depends on the Creator. Life is presented as a treasured divine blessing, a supreme earthly good. Male and female sexuality is viewed as a special gift and blessing, a sharing in God's prerogative to create human life: 'and God blessed them, and God said to them, "Be fruitful and multiply, and fill the earth"' (Gen. 1:28). The fact that the human being is a corporeal and spiritual being is of primary significance in Christian human anthropology. Empirical sciences are indispensable in their affirmation of the corporeal identity of the human person. The human body forms part of the visible world of matter, with which the human sciences are concerned. However, the body is more than the physical and biological life of the organism. As Molina states (de Dios Vial Correa & Sgreccia, 1998: 103), 'The strong anthropology of the tradition of Christian thought affirms that man is a person, endowed with a spiritual soul, by which he transcends matter and its limits and attains to the world of the spirit.' However, in contemporary science, the human soul becomes extrinsic to the body and ultimately irrelevant in preference to that which is able to be empirically quantified. The spiritual soul, not quantifiable by such scientific data, is dismissed and a disembodied dualistic notion of the human person permeates the culture. Such scientific reductionism of the human person is manifested in the contemporary discourse about the beginnings of human life, whereby the primacy of the technological imperative is the principle triumph of science. Such reductive methods of human science present human life merely in terms of mathematical expressions or hypothetical premises. Supported by moral pluralism, any truths regarding the common good that should be at the foundation of society are equivocally based on what is quantifiable or empirically justifiable. The body-subject has become the primary manifest of contemporary secular philosophical anthropology, and corporeality is the universally accepted expression of what it is to be a human being.

Ancient Greek philosopher Aristotle has strongly influenced scholars in their expression of the key tenets of human anthropology. For Aristotle, the earliest form of human life is from the first moment of ensoulment, whereby the soul proper to the human species is present (Lucas, 1998). The human embryo therefore would be destined from conception to bring to maturity what is already present: an individual of the human species with an embodied soul. Essentially, for Aristotle, 'it' would never be made human if it was not human from the very beginning. In the *Generation of Animals Book V (1)*, Aristotle states:

> when we are dealing with definite and ordered products of Nature, we must not say each is of a certain quality because it becomes so, but rather that they become so and so because they are so and so, for the process of Becoming or development attends upon Being and is for the sake of Being, not vice versa (Aristotle, cited in Ford, 1991).

Compatible with Aristotle's thought, in *Summa Theologica* St Thomas Aquinas defined human nature as the substantial composition of prime matter and the substantial spiritual form (Aquinas, ST, 1948, q75, q76, q90.) The human body is therefore a unity of body and soul, which presents the true nature of the human person. As human corporeality begins at the moment of conception, the metaphysical theme of the human person specific to Christian anthropology would also support the scientific truth about the early embryonic origins of human life. Present in every human life is the intention of the Creator that all humans participate in the mystery of the Incarnation, that God became flesh and dwelt among us (John 1:1–4) in the embodied person of Jesus Christ. The understanding of the theological status of the human embryo therefore presents that each human life at the earliest form is the first stage of human development as part of God's plan, and is a stage that is accomplished in human development through the Incarnation of Christ.

Other monotheistic religions support aspects of Christian anthropology on the moral status of the human embryo. Jewish and Islamic moral theologies have articulated slightly different positions on the understanding of when human life does begin. Each tradition has nuanced variances among its own scholars and religious teachers on such positions, but there are main premises that are accepted by most in each tradition. Jewish moral theology is pronatalist in orientation, and so places some restrictions on termination of pregnancy, highlighting that human life in utero has a sense of the sacred (Kurjak et al., 2007). In the Talmudic tradition, the foetus is formed at a certain stage of the pregnancy, that being 40 days for a male child and 80 days for a female child following conception (Jones, 2004). Interpretation of Jewish moral law relating to the moral status of the early stages of embryonic life varies depending upon the teaching source; however, it could be argued that a consistent position is that the embryo less than 40 days old does not hold the same moral status as the foetus. It is the relationship of the unborn to the mother that is the primary determinant if there are to be restrictions placed on any interventions that may limit the natural course of pregnancy (Kurjak et al., 2007).

In the Islamic tradition, human beings are given moral status by God during gestation, but not from conception. Ensoulment occurs from 40 to 120 days after conception, and therefore moral status is attributed only to the growing foetus and not the embryo (Kurjak et al., 2007). Ghaly (2012) affirms this position regarding a period of ensoulment of the embryo and foetus, but presents an argument that there is greater conferring of a sense of sacredness in human life at this point. Ghaly does not dismiss that this same sense may also be conferred earlier than 40 days after gestation. However, he does state that there is unanimous agreement among Islamic scholars that the fertilised ovum has no sanctity conferred until uterine implantation. Polytheistic traditions such as Hinduism and Buddhism characterise a general prohibition against doing harm to other human beings, including the unborn. For Hinduism, conscious awareness emerges during the fifth month of gestation, and so prior to that moral status is not conferred on the embryo or early developing foetus.

It is also important to note that not all Christian religious traditions hold the dogmatic position of the Catholic Church on the moral status of the human embryo, with a vast divergence among Protestant, Evangelical, Lutheran and Orthodox positions. Even within the Catholic Church, there has been opposition to the formal doctrinal positions on the sanctity of human life, the moral status of the embryo and the unborn, and the use of contraceptives to prevent pregnancy. Following the promulgation of *Humane Vitae* in 1968, Pope Paul

VI faced significant criticism from some Catholic theologians for the positions affirmed in this encyclical on the moral status of unborn human life and the prohibition of the use of contraceptives and abortion to regulate fertility (Curran, 2006). Theologians Tom Burns, Richard McCormack and Charles Curran were all vocal dissenters of *Human Vitae*, with Curran composing a statement critical of the ecclesiology and methodology of the pronouncements in the encyclical. Curran's statement was signed by over 600 theologians and other academics in the hope that there would be a reversal in the key teachings presented. This petition led to two schools of thought on such matters, a division that could be argued is still present in the twenty-first century in predominantly Western ecclesial sectors of the Catholic Church (Curran, 2006).

The emergence of the feminist movement in Western cultures during the 1960s saw increasing political lobbying for a woman's right to control reproduction, with unfettered access to abortion being one of the key goals of this movement. During this time, a key philosophical argument defending abortion was presented by feminist ethicist Judith Jarvis Thompson. In a seminal article titled 'A Defense of Abortion', Jarvis Thompson (1971) presented an argument that the growing embryo and foetus use a woman's body in a sort of opportunistic nature, treating the woman as a means to their own end of coming to birth. It is important to place this article by Jarvis Thompson in a historical timeframe. In the United States, the landmark legal decision of *Roe vs Wade*, which affirmed the preservation of women's rights, personal freedom and privacy with relation to reproductive choice was still two years away. In Australia, a Supreme Court ruling in 1969 by Justice Meinhennet stipulated that an abortion was not 'unlawful' if a doctor believed that the abortion was necessary to preserve the woman's life or her physical or mental health, and that this abortion could occur at any phase of the woman's pregnancy (De Crespigny & Savulescu, 2004). Radical feminism and the liberation movement are key features of this period of history, with relationships between men and women deeply politicised. Feminist scholars primarily argued that a woman's sexuality was disconnected from the social obligations of marriage and motherhood. In this period of social and political change, Jarvis Thompson's essay became one of the first academic scholarly articles to present a philosophical discussion that articulated a moral defence for abortion.

Throughout her discussion, Jarvis Thompson presents several analogies to frame the question of whether the woman has a moral obligation to sustain the life of the unborn foetus when this conflicts with her right to self-determination over what happens to her body. This article by Jarvis Thompson is one of the most frequently cited as a defence of the woman's right over that of an unborn child in the moral decision-making process that may lead to abortion. Two decades after Jarvis Thompson's article, another seminal paper that has strongly influenced the debate on the moral status of the embryo was published by English Baroness Mary Warnock. Civil libertarian Warnock's essay, 'Do Human Cells Have Rights?' (1987) was published in the first edition of the prestigious journal *Bioethics*. This article focused on human rights, and extended the debate about the moral and legal status of the earliest phases of human life. Warnock affirmed that, 'The right of the embryo, therefore, cannot be an actual right underpinned by actual law . . . [and] in a pluralistic society like our own, there do not exist uniform or universal moral sentiments.' (1987: 5, 9). Of significance in Warnock's essay is her use of the term 'pre-embryo' (an abbreviation for the term 'pre-implantation embryo'); it was one of the first academic papers to coin the term. The pre-embryo, she argues, is the period of time that human experimentation on a human embryo is morally permissible, being up to 14 days before the formation of the primitive streak. Warnock appeals to the empiricism of science to defend a rights discourse that rejects conferral of moral status to the earliest phase of human life, the embryo. This concept was developed after the advent of in-vitro fertilisation (IVF), and the issues it raised regarding the moral status of the embryo, including the wish to conduct research on in-vitro embryos.

To this point in the chapter, the focus has predominantly been upon exploring a theological and philosophical approach to the question of when human life begins. The following will now present a scientific analysis and discussion of this question. The term 'embryo' is derived from a Greek word meaning 'growing within' – that being the offspring growing in the womb. Biologically, the term 'embryo' usually refers to development from fertilisation up to the first eight completed weeks, after which the term 'foetus' is used. All somatic cells are derived from the fertilised egg through the process of mitosis, which produces two genetically identical daughter cells. A fertilised egg and its cell progeny require 42 mitotic divisions to supply the somatic cells for the development of a foetus to term. Only five more divisions suffice to provide the millions of cells needed for an adult (Liggins, 1982). While we do not have the exact time sequence for in vivo fertilisation, we do know the sequence for human fertilisation can be observed in vitro (Sathananthan, Trounson & Wood, 1986). Soon after the penetration of the sperm head into the egg's cytoplasm, the egg is activated and the paternal chromosomes de-condense within a new envelope to form the male pro-nucleus, while a membrane also develops around the remaining 23 female chromosomes to form the female pro-nucleus. During the next six to ten hours, the male and female pro-nuclei gradually move towards each other. During the pro-nuclear stage, DNA synthesis occurs in the chromosomes, resulting in each chromosome replicating itself to form two identical chromatin threads. The pro-nuclei come together some 16 hours after insemination. About 22 hours after insemination, syngamy occurs when the membranes of the two pro-nuclei begin to break down, allowing the male and female chromosomes to mingle, thereby completing fertilisation with the formation of a new diploid cell with its own unique genotype (Sathananthan, Trounson & Wood, 1986). This new cell is called a zygote because it yokes together the maternal and paternal chromosomes into one genetically new cell. After about two hours, its 23 pairs of homologous chromosomes line up for the onset of the first mitotic cleavage into two identical daughter cells.

The fundamental building block of a human body is the cell. Every cell, excluding gametes, beginning from the zygote, is diploid, and normally has 46 intermingling maternal and paternal chromosomes bonded into a nucleus. After these mix at syngamy, the zygote begins and is constituted into a genetically unique cell with its own diploid complement of 46 chromosomes. After both sets of chromosomes have mixed at syngamy, they are jointly organised to constitute a new human life. From then on, the diploid nucleus is the control panel for the life and destiny of its entire cell progeny, each of which is likewise normally diploid. Its newly constituted genetic code suffices to provide the internal central organisation required for the human being to develop to adulthood. Human life could not begin before the first basic building block of the human body with its unique genotype is actually constituted into the viable zygote, the first cell of a new human being (Ford, 2002). The completion of this union indicates that the zygote has been formed with its newly established genotype. As soon as it is constituted, the zygote begins to organise the first mitotic division of one cell into two identical daughter cells. This is quite significant inasmuch as the activity of organising cell division shows a new cell has already been formed and is functioning as such once the two pro-nuclei merge and their chromosomes become locked into an inherent life-principle. Sperm entry alone into the egg's cytoplasm is no more the beginning of the life-principle of a human embryo than the mixing of hydrogen and oxygen molecules in a container alone suffices to make a drop of water without a spark to activate their reaction to form water (Ford, 2002).

There is an in-built teleology and organisation in both sperm and egg to form a zygote. This teleology and organisation remain in the sperm's chromosomes and egg after the sperm is engulfed into the egg's cytoplasm. However, it is not until syngamy that their purpose is actually achieved, when a new diploid cell begins to exist. The zygote has now incorporated the genetic information of both gametes into its own distinct central organisation, thereby generating the beginning of a genetically new human life – a human being (Ford, 2002). As a result of the natural process of fertilisation, egg and sperm transcend themselves when they fuse and become a new diploid cell – a developing single cell zygote, the beginning of a new human life. The zygote divides to become a two-cell embryo and subsequently a four- and eight-cell embryo, and so on. The five- to seven-day-old embryo is called the blastocyst as it develops into a hollow ball of cells. Its outer layer of cells surrounding the inner cell mass (ICM) is called the trophoblast, the cell progeny of which give rise to the placenta. The cell progeny of the ICM in turn form the blastocyst, which implants in the uterus from days 6 to 13 after fertilisation (Ford, 2002).

An embryo is totipotent because it has the natural actual potential to form a body plan and entire offspring, including placental tissues. An isolated cell from a two-or even a four-cell embryo may also be totipotent. A sperm or an egg is not an embryo, but they have the potential to become an embryo once they fuse and form a zygote (Ford, 2011). In doing so, they become what they previously were not. With the completion of fertilisation, the embryo's unique genome is constituted, and directs human development throughout life. The genetic information encoded in the genes and chromosomes programs and coordinates integrated differentiation into various types of cells, tissues, structures and organs in a continuous, coordinated biological process, given a favourable uterine environment. Though the embryo depends on the mother for its continued life, it is independent of the mother with regard to the genetic information required for orderly development to birth and beyond (Ford, 1991). To be alive implies being able to live. A suitable environment like the uterus does not confer life, but enables a living embryo and foetus to continue to live (Ford, 2011).

It is important to note that every living or developing human embryo has the actual capacity of an integrated and functioning human organism. The presence of the human genome and its functioning is essential for an embryo to begin. Therefore, it is scientifically and philosophically credible to hold that the normal uni-directional and continuous biological development and growth suffice to establish the zygote as the one and same living being as the future human adult (Ford, 2011). Ford argues that 'the zygote may be regarded as an actual human individual and not merely a potential human individual in much the same way as an infant is an actual human being with potential to develop to maturity and adulthood' (2011: 324). In virtue of the creation of the spiritual (immaterial) soul within the emerging embryonic human being, it is credible to hold that a natural human person begins once the embryonic human individual is formed. Hence the spiritual soul would account for the human individual's rational nature and personhood from the completion of syngamy (Ford, 2011).

The Catholic Church has drawn on empirical science to add to the discussion and affirmation of its moral position that human life begins at conception, and that any action that intentionally harms the natural progression of this earliest form of human life is morally evil. One of the most definitive statements to the moral inviolability of the human embryo was given by the bishops of the Second Vatican Council. *Gaudium et Spes* (Pope Paul VI, 1965, n. 51) affirms that 'Life must be protected with the utmost care from the moment of conception; abortion and infanticide are abominable crimes.' The Church affirms in *Donum Vitae* that 'the zygote is the cell produced by the fusion of two gametes' (Congregation for the Doctrine of the Faith (CDF), 1987). As there is no empirical evidence for the moment when a soul is created for the human embryo, the Church states that even 'supposing a later animation, there is still nothing less than a human life, preparing for and calling for a soul in which the nature received from parents is completed' (CDF, 1974). Therefore, the developing human embryo is duly attributed human dignity and the moral inviolability of adults. The Declaration on Procured Abortion also affirms that:

> In the Middle Ages when the opinion was generally held that the spiritual soul was not present until after a few weeks, a distinction was made in the evaluation of the sin and the gravity of the penal sanctions ... But it was never denied at that time that procured abortion, even during the first few days, was objectively a grave sin. (CDF, 1974)

The Declaration on Procured Abortion also argues that fertilisation marks the beginning of the process of generation. It condemned the practice of direct abortion and the use of abortifacient and contraceptive methods to avoid pregnancy. The Declaration stated:

> From the time that the ovum is fertilised, a life is begun which is neither that of the father nor that of the mother; it is rather the life of a 'new living human being' – *novi vivientis humani* – with his own growth. It would never be made human if it were not human already ... From a moral point of view this is certain: even if a doubt existed concerning whether the fruit of conception is already a human person, it is objectively a grave sin to dare to risk murder. (CDF, 1974)

Although the Church holds that human life begins at fertilisation, the Declaration on Procured Abortion admits that it does not formally address the issue of when ensoulment occurs, and of when the fruit of conception becomes a person. It assumes that a human person begins at conception but the Church does not formally teach this.

From the promulgations of Vatican II to *Humane Vitae* from Pope Paul VI, various statements from the Congregation of the Doctrine of the Faith and Pope John Paul II's *Evangelium Vitae: The Gospel of Life*, the Catholic Church has constantly reaffirmed its centuries-held position that human life is sacred, and any attacks on human life from conception to a natural death constitute a grave moral evil. Pope John Paul II (1995, n 53) affirmed that 'Human life is sacred because from its beginning it involves "the creative action of God" and it remains forever in a special relationship with the Creator, who is its sole end. God alone is the Lord of life from its beginning until its end.' He also added that 'the Church has always taught and continues to teach that the result of human procreation, from the first moment of its existence, must be guaranteed unconditional respect . . . The human being is to be respected and treated as a person from the moment of conception.' (Pope John Paul II, 1995, n 60). Such pronouncements have resulted in criticism being directed at the Church from within its own theological and philosophical scholarship, as well as from secular ethicists and social commentators. Similarly, in an increasingly secular society, language that has no reference to religious moral traditions has become prominent in ethical and legal discourse on the issue of the origins of human life. However, it could also be argued that such over-emphasis on the use of biotechnical language to define when human life begins is problematic due to its moral ambiguity. Terms such as pre-embryo status, syngamy, primitive streak formation and foetal viability – contemporary positions on the moral status of the human embryo in utero, in vitro or in chemical suspension – have resulted in a reduction in arguments to those that focus predominantly on the potentiality of the embryo. The understanding that there is a continuity of an organism in the early phases of normal embryonic development, and that with a determined human trajectory a known embodied process will manifest, is rarely articulated in such scientific discourse.

This scientific language specific to human embryology has strongly influenced Australian legal definitions of the early origins of human life. In 2002, a new Australian federal law presented a different position on the legal status of the human embryo. In the *Research Involving Human Embryos Act 2002* (Cth), the following legal definition is provided:

human embryo means a discrete entity that has arisen from either:

(a) The first mitotic division when fertilisation of a human oocyte by a sperm is complete;

or

(b) Any other process that initiates organised development of a biological entity when a human nuclear genome or altered human nuclear genome that has the potential to develop up to, or beyond, the stage at which the primitive streak appears;

And has not yet reached 8 weeks of development since the first mitotic division

The theistic notion that the human embryo is due respect and protection as being at the earliest stage of human life is challenged by this 2002 Australian law. Scientific research on human embryos is legally permissible in Australia up until the formation of the primitive streak in the in-vitro embryo, which occurs at 14 days after fertilisation. At this point, science affirms that the embryo could no longer split into more than one embryo, therefore this phase of the human embryo's development marks its individuality. However, an argument against this position is that the embryo is no different before or after the formation of the primitive streak. As American medical ethicist and obstetrician Patrick Yeung (2005: 70) states, 'Nothing is added, and nothing is taken away. The appearance of the primitive streak, or its clinical marker implantation is not the beginning of human life.' The primitive streak actually provides confirmation that an embodied process is continuing along a scientifically confirmed trajectory – the normal embryonic develop-ment of human life. The teleology manifested in the pre-determined devel-opmental process from an embryo to a newborn baby and eventual adult argues that the human being must somehow be present in the zygote from the constitution of its unique genome (Ford, 2008, 2011). The ontological char-acter of this ongoing teleological causal influence on the developing embryo generates solid and reasonable grounds for holding that the human zygote is the same living being as the growing embryo, foetus, newborn child and adult human being. These considerations, coupled with the continuity of human development from the zygote, with its inbuilt ontological relations, provide credible scientific and philosophical reasons in support of the zygote being a human being, a natural person (Ford, 2008, 2011).

Contemporary biological sciences recognise that an organism is an independent, embodied process that actively follows a particular trajectory. Yeung (2005) argues that the organism created in the beginning from gametic human origins can therefore only be human, and that such a trajectory follows an independent, embodied process. Ford (2007: 18) supports this position in stating:

> Each newly formed zygote is endowed with its own unique genome which functions as a live blueprint. There are obvious indicators of purpose, finalism and direction in the interactions of cells, the formation of a human body plan and the orderly development of tissues and organs to achieve this end. Respect for human embryos is based on the divinely conferred natural actual potential of their genome, given a suitable environment, to direct and organise continuous development and growth from conception to birth and to adulthood.

Philosophical reasoning also supports this position. The teleology or finalism manifested in the developmental process from the embryo to a newborn infant provides grounds for arguing that the human being must be present in the zygote from its constitution. The ontological character of this ongoing teleological causal influence in the developing embryo provides good grounds for accepting that the human zygote is the same living being as the foetus, newborn child and adult human being. These considerations suffice to provide credible scientific and philosophical reasons in support of the first cell, the zygote, being deemed a human being, a natural person (Ford, 2008; Ford, 2011: 324). Human nature enables human embryos to develop to the stage where, without ceasing to be the same living beings, they can exercise rationally self-conscious and free acts. Really, there is no justification for the reductionism that views embryonic human life – naturally or artificially conceived – as no more than genetic products, devoid of significance and value. From a theistic perspective, the formative process and the fruit of human generation have a claim to unconditioned moral respect (Ford, 1991).

From a scientific, ethical, social, legal and cultural perspective, the question of when a human life begins has differing interpretations in contemporary society. This chapter has provided a brief analysis of some of these key arguments, focusing on the theological and philosophical foundations of the Catholic Church's position that human life begins at conception. The science of embryology has been appealed to in order to present an argument that the origins of human life are indeed from conception, and therefore it is credible to hold that a natural human person begins once the embryonic human individual is formed.

Reflective exercises

13.1 What are the main features of a Christian human anthropology, and how do these relate to the question of when human life begins?

13.2 Summarise some of the other theistic traditions' positions on when human life begins. What implications does this have for assisted reproductive technologies (ARTs), embryonic stem cell research, termination of pregnancy in the first trimester and human cloning?

13.3 What is the significance of the 'pre-embryo' phase of human development as highlighted by Baroness Mary Warnock in her article 'Do Human Cells Have Rights?'? Do you think that there is such a phase in embryonic development? What is your moral and/or scientific foundation for this position?

13.4 Summarise the scientific development of the earliest phase of human life as described in the work of Ford, referenced in this chapter. What is the significance of the embryonic period of syngamy, the primitive streak and twinning to the ethical question of when human life begins? How do these terms connect to contemporary Australian law?

13.5 The commencement of this chapter presented a discussion about the controversial 2012 article 'After Birth Abortion: Why Should the Baby Live?' by Australian medical ethicists Alberto Giubilini and Francesca Minerva. This article can be accessed via an online data search. Review the article and present ethical arguments that support or refute the claims made by the authors. Review utilitarian, natural law, feminist, libertarian and Kantian ethical reasoning to formulate your arguments and conclusions.

References

Aquinas, T. (1948). *Summa Theologica*, trans. Fathers of the Dominican Province. New York: Benziger Brothers.

Aristotle (1963). *Generation of Animals*, trans. A. L. Peck & M. A. London. Cambridge, MA: Harvard University Press.

Congregation for the Doctrine of the Faith (CDF) (1974). Declaration on procured abortion. Retrieved 21 October 2014 from <http://www.vaitcan.va>.

—— (1987). *Donum vitae. Instruction on respect for human life in its origin and on the dignity of procreation replies to* certain questions of the day. Retrieved 21 October 2014 from <http://www.vatican.va>.

Curran, C. (2006). *Loyal dissent: Memoirs of a Catholic theologian*. Washington, DC: Georgetown University Press.

De Crespigny, L. J. & Savulescu, J. (2004). Abortion: Time to clarify Australia's confusing laws. *Medical Journal of Australia*, 181(4): 201–3.

de Dios Vial Correa, J. & Sgreccia, E. (1998). *Identity and statute of human embryo: Proceedings. Documenti Vaticani. Volume 3 of Proceedings of the Assembly of the Pontifical Academy for Life, Pontificia Academia pro Vita (Roma)*. Charlottesville, VA: University of Virginia.

Ford, N. (1991). *When did I begin? Conception of the human individual in history, philosophy and science*. Cambridge: Cambridge University Press.

—— (2002). *The prenatal person: Ethics from conception to birth*. Oxford: Blackwell.

—— (2007). Moral respect due to the human embryo. *Ethics Education*, 13(1): 13–20.

—— (2008). Interview with Norman Ford. *Monash Bioethics Review*, 27(3): 25–33.

—— (2011). A Catholic ethical perspective on human reproductive technology. In J. G. Schenker (ed.), *Ethical dilemmas in assisted reproductive technologies*. Berlin: Walter de Gruyter.

Ghaly, M. (2012). Islam, paternity and the beginning of life. *Zygon*, 47(1): 175–213.

Giubilini, A. & Minerva, F. (2012). After-birth abortion: Why should the baby live? *Journal of Medical Ethics*, 39(5): 261–3.

Jarvis Thompson, J. (1971). A defense of abortion. *Philosophy and Public Affairs*, 1(1): 47–66.

Jones, D. A. (2004). *The soul of the embryo: An enquiry into the status of the human embryo in the Christian tradition*. London: Continuum.

Kuhse, H. & Singer, P. (1988). *Should the baby live? The problem of handicapped infants*. Oxford: Oxford University Press

—— (1990). Individuals, humans and persons: The issue of moral status. In P. Singer, H. Kuhse, S. Buckle, K. Dawson & P. Kasimba, *Embryo experimentation*. Cambridge: Cambridge University Press.

Kurjak, A., Carrera, J. M., McCullough, L. B. & Chervenak, F. A. (2007). Scientific and religious controversies about the beginning of human life: The relevance of the ethical concept of the fetus as a patient. *Journal of Perinatal Medicine*, 35(5): 376–83.

Liggins, G. C. (1982). Fetal growth. In C. R. Austin & R. V. Short (eds), *Embryonic and fetal development: Book 2, reproduction in mammals*, Cambridge: Cambridge University Press.

Lucas. R. (1998). The anthropological status of the human embryo. In *Identity and Status of the Human Embryo: Proceedings of the Third*

Assembly of the Pontifical Academy
for Life; Pontifical Academia pro
Vita (Roma). Charlottesville, VA:
University of Virginia.

Pope John Paul II (1995). *Evangelium
Vitae: The gospel of life.* Retrieved
21 October 2014 from <http://
www.vatican.va>.

Pope Paul VI (1965). *Gaudium et Spes.
Pastoral constitution of the Church in
the modern world.* Retrieved 21
October 2014 from <http://www.
vatican.va>.

*Research Involving Human Embryos Act
2002* (Cth).

Sathananthan, A. H., Trounson, A. O. &
Wood, C. (1986). *Atlas of fine
structure of human sperm, eggs and
embryos cultured in vitro.*
Philadelphia, PA: Praeger.

Singer, P. (1993). *Practical ethics.*
(2nd ed.). Cambridge: Cambridge
University Press.

Warnock, M. (1987). Do human cells
have rights? *Bioethics,* 1(1): 1–14.

Yeung, P. (2005). When does human life
begin? *RedOrbit.* Retrieved 20
September 2014 from <http://www.
redorbit.com/news/science/189217/
when_does_human_life_begin>

14 Autonomy and consent

Jānis (John) Ozoliņš

One the most vexed questions in healthcare involves patient autonomy, and the extent to which patients are able to make decisions about their healthcare. It may not always be the case that patients will be able to understand the information that they have been given and decide what advice regarding their treatment they should follow. The question of autonomy and the extent to which patients are able to give informed consent to the treatment being recommended to them becomes more difficult as their health deteriorates. These issues will be explored in this chapter.

The idea that patients need to be asked to consent to the medical and healthcare treatment that is being proposed to them is reasonably modern. After all, the healthcare practitioner is the professional, the person with the expertise to decide what treatments are needed by the patient in order to return to health. If a patient needs an operation to remove a tumour, they are expected to accept the surgeon's advice and have the operation. The Hippocratic Oath states nothing about asking patients for their informed consent before the physician prescribes medication or performs surgery. Despite this, it has generally become accepted that, because patients are autonomous, self-determining human persons, they need to be fully informed of the treatment options available to them, and to decide, having assessed the available information and taken appropriate advice, what treatments they will undertake. This is the recognition that a pathway to health will involve the active participation of patients – that is, it is not simply a matter of patients passively receiving treatment. The whole person needs to be involved in recovery to full health.

This means that one of the most important matters with which healthcare practitioners need to deal is ensuring that patients are able to make an informed decision about their treatment. Although, superficially, one might think that there is nothing simpler than asking patients whether they understand the nature of a particular health problem they are suffering and the treatment proposed, the situation is rather more complex. In this chapter, we will consider the following issues:

- why we need to seek informed consent
- what is meant by autonomy and informed consent
- what information should be given to patients
- what is meant by voluntary consent, and
- how we assess the competence of the patient to give consent.

We will also briefly discuss what is meant by risk in relation to explaining the benefits and harms of treatments to patients, and consider different ways in which consent might be established. Finally, we will briefly discuss the provision of consent by minors.

Why seek informed consent?

There is a very large body of literature that addresses the question of informed consent, which has particular importance in medical and other health-related treatment, as well as in healthcare research and clinical trials. It is not, however, restricted to these contexts, but is of importance in other kinds of disciplinary areas. Teachers, psychologists, sociologists, paediatricians and others working with children, for example, have particular responsibilities in seeking not just parental consent, but also the assent of children when they wish to treat them or involve them in research. The seeking of informed consent is recognition that the respect we owe persons obliges us to involve them as far as possible in decisions that affect their lives. Its significance is evident in every walk of life: downloading a simple application (or app) on a smartphone always comes with a list of terms and conditions that those downloading must accept before they can access the app. Often these conditions will include statements in relation to data that is collected about the user of the application and how that data may be used. Often this data relates to questions of privacy and to third parties who might have access to the collected data. Whether people actually read these terms and conditions is another matter, and if they do not, then their consent is hardly informed. Nevertheless, it is the case that consent to these is required before the app can be downloaded and used. Problems arise when there is insufficient information provided in relation to apps and people are misled.

In general, most people in the Western world are familiar with being asked to accept the terms and conditions for the use of goods and services. Although acceptance of terms and conditions is a form of consent, in many instances it is done without careful reading of them, and acceptance is simply regarded as another step in the download process. Consent is voluntary, but that is all. In healthcare, however, consent needs to be not only voluntary, but also informed, since an individual's health is a much more serious matter than the downloading of an app. Moreover, within the healthcare field, many countries acknowledge that the autonomy of human beings demands that, as far as possible, they should make decisions concerning their healthcare themselves. *The International Code of Medical Ethics* of the World Medical Association (2006) explicitly states that a physician will respect a competent patient's right to accept or refuse treatment.

Informed consent from patients is sought for a number of reasons:

- It has become accepted practice for patients to be asked about their treatment and to consent to it.
- Respect for persons demands that we involve them in decision-making about their treatment.
- Patients are autonomous, self-determining individuals, and this entails that they make their own decisions about their welfare.
- There are legal questions about any data that might be collected about patients, and how it is to be used. There are risks involved in all treatment, and patients need to know about these.
- Holistic treatment involves cooperation between patients and healthcare professionals to ensure that the treatments received by patients will be likely to lead to better health.

This list of reasons is not exhaustive, but it is evident that seeking informed consent from patients can be justified on a number of different grounds.

Some objections

Although we do not intend to address all of the issues that arise in relation to informed consent, it is evident that the assumption that all patients are independent rational thinkers who are able to fully understand and make a considered decision in relation to their treatment is questionable. The supposition that patients will somehow understand what the heathcarers are trying to do is in many cases quite false. This is most apparent in complex treatment, where patients are unlikely to have a sufficiently strong healthcare background themselves to adequately assess the likely outcomes of treatment – especially if this involves comparing alternative treatments. Onora O'Neill (2004) argues that, despite the great emphasis that is placed on autonomy, trust in medical and healthcare practitioners has fallen. Trust, she argues, has not received the same attention as autonomy. For example, a woman may have a prolapsed uterus and, depending on the medical assessment provided of the seriousness of the prolapse, a range of treatments may be proposed, ranging from surgery to pelvic floor exercises. It is difficult to see how she can make an informed judgement about what advice to accept in relation to treatment, and from whom, without fully understanding the pros and cons of each treatment. To a large degree, she will need to place her trust in the team of healthcarers that is treating her.

Another stark example is provided by considering the issues of living donor donation of organs or tissues. For instance, consenting to donate a kidney to a relative is a very difficult decision, only partly made easier by the donor's evident desire to help a close relative. In such a case, a parent might have no qualms about donating a kidney to a child if it would save that child. This situation, however, might change if the potential donor is informed that her other kidney is diseased and removal of the healthy kidney would in a very short time result in kidney failure and the need to be placed on dialysis. It would be further complicated if the donor is a sole parent with four other children depending on her continuing to support them for quite some time into the future. In addition, emotions may also cloud judgement, especially in cases involving the health and welfare of children. It is clear that informed consent involves some very complex decision-making, and raises the question of the competence of individuals directly affected by treatments to actually give voluntary informed consent.

Corrigan (2003) argues that although most people agree that informed consent ought to be obtained, it is not obvious how meaningful consent is given. This is because particular understandings of freedom and autonomy may mean that there are different conceptions of what is meant by consent, let alone informed consent, and so the choices that are offered by the healthcare professional might be premised on a different understanding from that of the patient. Though Corrigan argues her case from within a bioethical framework, the argument has more general applicability. Thus, in certain cultures, consent is not a matter for an individual since the idea of autonomy being an attribute of an individual is simply foreign. Freedom and autonomy are much more closely tied to the community to which the individual belongs, so a decision about whether to undergo a particular treatment is not one that the individual (as understood within the Western tradition) would contemplate making. Although, according to a Western perspective, such a view of individuality as perhaps being invested in the clan or tribal group seems to result in a reduction of freedom to make choices, a different perspective would see it as sparing the individual from making decisions alone. It is therefore possible that a different conception of freedom might determine a different outcome.

Autonomy

At first glance, when we think about the concept of autonomy it appears to be quite straightforwardly a synonym for independence, self-sufficiency and sovereignty. Typically, in relation to persons, autonomy is defined as the capacity to think, decide and, on the basis of reflective, rational thought and decision, act freely and independently. Autonomy means that persons are able to control their own lives, because they are free to make their own decisions and to choose their own actions – even if a majority of other people disagree with their decisions and actions. In Western liberal thought, autonomy is taken to be the most important value and, as a consequence, a plurality of values and beliefs are tolerated, so that there is little public consensus about core moral values (Charlesworth, 1993). This lack of consensus also applies to autonomy itself, and a range of opinion exists about the extent to which human beings can be independent, self-sufficient and sovereign – a law unto themselves (Gillon, 1985).

Autonomy can be understood as having at least seven attributes (Rendtorff, 2008). These are:

- being able to independently create ideas and goals for life
- having self-control and a developed moral understanding
- freely engaging in rational decision-making and action
- taking personal responsibility for one's actions
- having control of one's destiny in relation to healthcare, and giving voluntary informed consent to treatments where required
- having respect for one's privacy and that of others, and
- taking one's responsibility to one's community seriously.

We do not intend to discuss these attributes in detail, as we are directly concerned with the connection of autonomy to informed consent; however, some general observations can be made. First, it is evident that the conception of autonomy is very specifically directed to human beings. Autonomy as it is described here will not be applicable to non-human animals; however, this does not mean that non-human animals cannot act autonomously in a more restricted sense. Second, the exercise of the attributes of autonomy is not disconnected from interaction with other human beings, since they imply that those in the community in which one lives will value autonomy for themselves and others. Paradoxically, we might say that autonomy implies dependence on others. Third, underlying the attributes of autonomy are other values, such as respect for persons, that support its exercise. Lastly, an interpretation of the attributes involves assumptions about what kinds of beings humans are.

Therefore, autonomy cannot be thought of in isolation from an understanding of the nature of human persons, their relationship with others and other values. First, we have to understand human persons as the kinds of beings who have inherent dignity, to whom respect is owed and who are to be treated as ends in themselves. Second, we need to recognise that autonomy is not an absolute value, and that there are limitations to the extent to which we can exercise autonomy. Third, autonomy is not the only value that is to be taken into account in decision-making about actions, whether in relation to healthcare or other areas of our lives. Our relationships with others, for example, may also play a part in our decision-making. Someone may choose to delay a hip replacement, for instance, because another member of their family needs their immediate care. In this case, the value given to care affects the exercise of autonomy in relation to the hip replacement operation.

Informed consent

Patients are asked to give informed consent, as we have seen, when they are faced with decisions about their healthcare treatment. They are also asked to give informed consent when medical and healthcare researchers invite them to be participants in their research projects. Although there are differences between how the conception of informed consent is applied in these separate contexts, what is meant by informed consent will be the same in both cases. Informed consent has four aspects:

- the provision of information
- the chance to deliberate over the information provided
- freedom to make a voluntary choice, and
- competence to make a choice.

All four of these elements must be present if patients are to give genuine informed consent. It is insufficient to simply provide information alone, but not enable patients to deliberate over the information, for example. Nor is it sufficient to give no information, but expect patients to make choices. It is a legal requirement in Australia to provide information to patients in relation to their health treatments and medical procedures, but it is also evident that they need to be capable of understanding what treatments they are to undergo and able to deliberate about them before giving consent (National Health and Medical Research Council, 2004).

What information needs to be given to patients?

It is evident that we need to give patients sufficient information that will enable them to give informed consent – this is notionally true. The difficult part is determining what information, and in what detail, is to be given so that patients are informed and, more importantly, have enough understanding of the treatments or procedures to be able to give consent. Patients cannot be considered to be informed if they are not told in understandable language what procedures or treatments they are to undergo, or if they are told only some of what they are to undergo. Obviously, once patients are actually admitted to hospital, they would have already discussed the procedures or treatments prior to admission, but the provision of information ought not to cease on admission. Patients still need to be informed about the details of what is to be done and to consent at each step. An anaesthetist, for example, will typically visit patients after they have been admitted. In providing information, the anaesthetist needs to detail all risks associated with anaesthesia and determine whether patients are allergic to particular drugs. Patients need to be alerted to possible adverse reactions, and to what to expect once the effects of the anaesthesia wear off (Australian and New Zealand College of Anaesthetists, 2005).

In general, then, included in the information that is provided to patients is an indication of the possible risks that might be involved in their treatment. It is almost impossible for there to be treatments that are completely free of any risk, since it is possible even in the most innocuous procedure for there to be an unexpected adverse reaction. In providing information, a balance needs to be struck between detailing every possible adverse reaction – no matter how remote the possibility may be – and not providing enough information.

Providing too much information can result in patients not reading or not comprehending what they are reading.

Healthcare professionals need to be aware of the context patients typically encounter when they are admitted to hospital. For example, patients are often admitted to surgery on the day of admission, and are processed by a succession of clerical, nursing and medical staff. They are expected to sign a number of forms while waiting for a bed to become available, and for visits from the surgeon and the anaesthetist. Hospitals are busy and noisy environments and, unless patients are themselves healthcare practitioners, these surroundings are both confronting and unfamiliar (Braun, Skene & Merry, 2010). As far as possible, patients need to be provided with information in an environment in which it is possible for them to exercise judgement in a calm and rational manner.

Voluntariness

Patients need to consent to treatments and procedures voluntarily. This does not just mean that it is simply a matter of asking for consent and taking ready agreement to be *prima facie* evidence for voluntariness. As Aristotle (1976) explains in the *Nichomachean Ethics*, the explication of voluntary action is no simple matter. For example, suppose – to use Aristotle's classic example – we are on a ship that is caught in a sudden storm and it is in danger of sinking unless its sailors are able to lighten the ship. This can be accomplished by throwing its cargo overboard. Of course, since the livelihood of the sailors depends on the cargo, this is not an action that they want to choose. Nevertheless, in order to save their lives, they decide to throw the cargo overboard. Do the sailors act voluntarily? Consider another example where a person swimming at a beach is caught by a strong undertow that sweeps them out to sea. The second case is an example of involuntariness, and the feature of the situation that enables us to draw this conclusion is that the swimmer had no choice: the force of the undertow was sweeping him out to sea. The first case is not so easy to classify as either voluntary or involuntary. It is evident that the storm has forced the sailors to do what they would not otherwise have done – namely, to throw their precious cargo overboard. On the other hand, the storm did not take away their ability to deliberate over the course of action that they should take. In being able to deliberate and to decide a course of action based on an analysis of the situation, we would say that the sailors acted voluntarily in throwing the cargo overboard.

Patients are in a similar situation to the sailors. They require some kind of treatment or procedure because of a particular ailment or medical condition. There is an element of involuntariness, since their ailment or condition compels them to seek treatment. The opportunity to deliberate over what action to take, however, introduces an element of voluntariness, and this is important. Aquinas, in commenting on Aristotle's example, agrees. There are features of involuntariness in the example, since no one throws cargo overboard unless there is a good reason to do so. Similarly, no one normally seeks medical treatment unless they have to. Voluntariness enters the equation when individuals are given sufficient information, have the opportunity to deliberate and can consent to treatments and procedures (Aquinas, 1948).

An aspect of actions that are involuntary is that they are actions done through ignorance. That is, an aspect of involuntariness is found in the case of a person who is ignorant of particular conditions about which, and on which, human activity is exercised, as Aristotle (1976) says. In particular, in this account of ignorance, we are interested in ignorance due not to insensibility caused by, say, inebriation, but rather that due to a lack of knowledge of the situation in which one is acting. That is to say, certain circumstances have not been made known to the agent determining to act. Thus, where clinicians want their patients to undergo particular treatments or procedures, an important element in enabling genuine informed consent is to ensure that the patients have sufficient knowledge and understanding of what is being requested.

Voluntariness crucially depends not just on healthcare professionals supplying detailed information about what is being requested, but on patients understanding what the information supplied means. Only then are they in a position to make a voluntary decision to undergo the proposed treatment or procedure. For patients, this means that the information must be pitched at their level of understanding. The practical result of this requirement is that the information supplied must be free of technical jargon and explain in relatively simple terms what the treatment or procedure involves, and the seriousness of the patient's condition. An aspect of this will also be drawing to the attention of patients the possible adverse effects of the treatments or procedures. For example, in an operation to drain fluid from the brain, a patient would need to be told about any risks of damage to the spinal cord and any possible side-effects following the surgery.

Competence of the participant

It is possible that no matter how carefully healthcare practitioners explain treatments and procedures, patients may not be competent to give informed consent. For example, there are certain kinds of mental impairments that might limit the capacity of persons to fully understand what is being asked of them, and hence they may not be able to competently give informed consent. Someone suffering from early Alzheimer's disease or another form of dementia, for instance, may seem to be competent, but because of various memory deficits, may be unable to make an informed decision. Other less obvious instances where there may be limited competence to make an informed decision to participate in research could be due to temporary impairments such as depression, bipolar disorder or simply tiredness. Some of these impairments may not be obvious to the treating clinician. Severe illness may also limit someone's capacity to give fully informed, voluntary consent.

Competence assumes that patients have not only read the information, but have understood what the implications of the procedures or treatments are. Often there are benefits to a particular treatment, but there can also be harms. An aggressive treatment regime, for example, may have the best prospects of beating a particular condition, but it may have side-effects that are unacceptable to a particular participant. Another, less aggressive, treatment may be preferable. Those treating patients need to be reasonably assured that they have understood the information they have been given, and are able to give informed consent.

Risk

Healthcare practitioners need to provide patients with information about the benefits of the proposed treatments or procedures, but also an estimate of the risk of their harms, should they consent to undergo them. Even in the most innocuous procedure, there is always the possibility of harm, so as far as possible, without creating alarm in the minds of patients, it is important to explain to them what the risks are. Obviously, if a procedure has little benefit but has significant potential for harm, it might not be wise for it to be undertaken. For example, undergoing labiaplasty for cosmetic reasons has little or no health benefit, since it is not undertaken to improve the function of the particular body part, but for appearance alone. The risk of harm, however, includes bleeding, loss of sensation, scarring and nerve damage (Moran & Lee, 2013). As a general rule, in treating patients, healthcare staff seek to minimise the harm they do and maximise the benefits of the treatment. Rather obviously, if a patient presents with an ingrown toenail, the physician does not immediately call for the amputation of the patient's foot. In this case, the harm clearly outweighs the benefit, but in many cases it is not so easy to determine whether there are genuine benefits to be had that justify the risk of harms. Cosmetic surgery is highly controversial, for example, because it is not always obvious that the risk of harm is less than the promised benefits.

In assessing risk, there are two variables that need to be considered: first, there are considerations of a likelihood of harm occurring; and second, there are considerations of the level of harm that the treatments or procedures will involve. Thus, if the procedure is such that it could result in death, it is at once seen that this would represent a catastrophic harm to the patient, even if the benefits were enormous. Though it might be thought that a such procedure should not be undertaken, it may be that the likelihood of such as catastrophic harm is very small, and so the risk is correspondingly small. In daily life, for example, there is a finite probability that when we drive our cars on the road we could be killed, but since the probability is small, we accept the risk associated with driving our cars. Similarly, travelling by plane enables us to reach far-off destinations in a matter of hours, but it is obvious that the harm to us should the engines fail is catastrophic, since death is a likely outcome. The probability of such a catastrophic event is low, but calculable nevertheless. In estimating risk in these cases, we first weigh up the benefits against the harms, and then calculate the likelihood of the harms coming about against the likelihood of the benefits coming about.

In assessing the risk to patients of proposed treatments, the clinician has to set out quite clearly what the possible risks are. That is, the kinds of harms that are anticipated outcomes of the treatments or procedures have to be enumerated and their probabilities estimated as accurately as possible. In general, treatments and procedures that result in a low risk of harm are preferred to those that have a high risk of harm. This does not mean that procedures or treatments that have a high risk of harm can never be undertaken – for example, a patient may be facing imminent death, but could be saved by a procedure that is itself highly risky. In such cases, physicians are required to reduce the extent of harms as far as possible. This may be done by ensuring that, in the eventuality of harms arising, there are plans in place to minimise the harm. For example, if in a particular intervention there is some possibility of, say, a heart attack, then the physician would be expected to anticipate this eventuality and have a medical team on stand-by to reduce the risk of an adverse event as far as possible.

Associated with the level of risk is the question of the competence of the healthcare practitioner to carry out the proposed treatment or procedure. In general, if what is to be undertaken is beyond the competence of the treating practitioner, then it ought not to be undertaken, since this clearly increases the risk of harm to the patient. For example, if a nurse has not been trained to change a pain-relief regimen for a patient, then that nurse should not give the patient an increased dose of a painkiller or additional medication, even if the nurse is requested by the patient to provide it. Patients cannot be put at risk because those treating them do not have: adequate training to provide the treatment; proper, reliable equipment; and sufficient skills to operate the equipment. With new and increasingly sophisticated equipment becoming available for various treatments and procedures, it is vital that healthcare practitioners upgrade their qualifications to maintain the skill levels required to operate medical equipment and to provide an excellent standard of care to patients.

Limits of consent

There are two aspects to the limiting of consent. First, consent by patients is generally given only for specific treatments and procedures, rather than for all treatments. A treating physician will need to ask for the consent of patients again if they decide that an existing treatment is not proving to be efficacious, needs to be discontinued and an alternative treatment should be proposed. Similarly, if the physician decides to supplement a treatment with another procedure, this will also require consent. For example, a patient may be being treated with radiotherapy for a cancer. If the treating physician decides that chemotherapy is also required, the patient will need to be informed and consent given for this treatment. Second, patients are always at liberty to withhold their consent, and decide not to undergo the proposed additional treatment. They can also decide to stop treatment altogether. In such cases, consent is limited to treatments that patients are prepared to undergo, knowing the full balance of benefits and risks that may occur through their participation.

Patients can normally withdraw their consent at any time, and this is something that healthcare practitioners need to be aware of and accept. Patients may decide that the treatment is burdensome and futile, and that they no longer wish to continue it. They may also decide on some other form of treatment from some other healthcare provider. Importantly, healthcare professionals need to be aware that consent at any stage is not permanent, but may need renegotiation at different points in the treatment. The relationship between practitioners and patients is a crucial part of the treatment process, and it should not be assumed by practitioners or patients that it does not require nurturing. Open communication between both parties is important to ensure that there is continued understanding of the progress of treatments and for the building of trust. Trust between patients and those treating them are vital if consent to treatments is to be maintained. Healthcare practitioners must ensure that they inform patients that, even though they may give consent in writing, it is understood that they may withdraw from treatment. Moreover, they will not suffer any penalty as a result of their withdrawal of consent. That is, if patients withdraw from a particular treatment, they should not receive less nursing attention than they otherwise would have received had they continued with participation.

Consent is limited too in cases where patients are incompetent, very ill, unconscious, very young, demented, very frail or perhaps only confused. In cases where patients are rushed to hospital for emergency treatment – for instance, if a patient is suffering a heart attack – it would be not only impractical to ask for informed consent for the treatment, but also life-threatening and negligent. Paramedics called to the scene of an accident may have only limited time to stabilise a patient, and seeking informed consent would simply be inappropriate. Of course, if the patient is conscious, this does not mean that what is going to be done ought not to be explained to the patient and their cooperation obtained. In other cases, patients may be confused and frail, and asking for informed consent could be very taxing for them, especially if there are complexities in their treatment. Obviously, those who are unconscious are unable to give consent and, in such cases, consent will need to be given by whoever is empowered to do so on their behalf. The same will apply in other cases where individuals are unable to give consent themselves.

Consent for those below the age of 18

In general, in Australian law, consent to medical treatment cannot be given by a minor, where a minor is defined as a person below the age of 18. This is because, as we have already said, informed consent is taken to mean that the persons have the capacity to understand the information they are being given, are able to deliberate and have the maturity to give free and uncoerced consent. Most obviously, babies and very young children will not have the capacity to give informed consent, but it is not quite so clear in the case of someone who is 17 years old. This is recognised in some state jurisdictions, such as New South Wales, where a child aged 14 years and over may consent to their own medical and dental treatment (*Minors (Property and Contracts) Act 1970* (NSW). Despite this, the Act also acknowledges that parents may give consent to medical and dental treatment to children under the age of 16. In practice, in cases of medical and dental treatments of minors below the age of 18, it would seem to be wise to not only seek consent from minors, where they are 14 and over, but also from parents and guardians. Indeed, it should be normal practice to ensure that, in all cases where the child is aged less than 18, they are fully informed and comprehend what is required of them through their participation in treatment or procedures. Willingness to assent to such treatment or procedures also needs to be supported by the consent of the minor's parents or guardians.

Asking children for their consent should not be restricted to any particular age group. As they develop, children are able to understand a great deal more than is sometimes thought. They should also be part of the consent process to the extent that they are able. It is nevertheless important that the healthcare practitioner does not assume that children will have the same understanding of what is being asked of them as an adult does. They need to be aware that, in order to gain consent from a child, they will need to explain everything in as simple a way as possible. This will, of course, vary according to the age of the child. In all cases, healthcare practitioners need to ensure that the environment in which a child is informed about the treatments or procedures provides for the child's physical safety, emotional and psychological security, and general well-being.

Consideration to the following should be given when seeking to involve minors in consent to treatments and procedures. Healthcare practitioners should be satisfied that:

- young persons are mature enough to understand the relevant information and to give consent, although vulnerable because of relative immaturity in other respects

- the consent from those responsible for the young person is also sought; for health professionals, consideration of relevant laws is also an important consideration
- the benefits outweigh the harms for the category of young persons to which they belong (for example, some procedures might not be suitable for very young children)
- where the young person is estranged or separated from parents or guardians, provision is made to protect the young person's safety, security and well-being in decision-making about treatments (in this case, the child's circumstances may mean they are at some risk – for example, because of being homeless).

Different ways of establishing consent

In most cases, the most appropriate way in which consent can be established is by asking the patient to complete a consent form. In accordance with the Australian *NHMRC General Guidelines for Medical Practitioners on Providing Information to Patients* (2004), a consent form should contain a clear statement of what treatments the patient is to undergo and anything they are required to do, such as fast or refrain from drinking alcohol or other activities. This means that it is not enough for the consent form to indicate that patients agree to their direct participation in such procedures or treatment. A written form is not the only means of seeking consent, although clearly there are cases where this is the best means of doing so, especially where serious life-threatening treatments and procedures are proposed. This, as we have already discussed in some detail, may not be sufficient, since patients may not understand the details of what they are being told. This means that very often matters on the form will need to be explained verbally.

Not every situation requires a written consent form. In many cases, it would be burdensome and unwieldy to use written consent. In such cases, verbal consent is sufficient. For example, a physiotherapist may be giving a relatively simple treatment on a limb – say, treatment of a muscular injury with ultrasound – for which a written consent form would be unnecessary, but consent to treatment would nevertheless need to be given. In some cases, where patients are of non-English speaking background, an interpreter might be required to explain the treatments or procedures. This would need to be done verbally.

A checklist to aid practitioners would also be helpful. For example:

- Do you understand the information that I have read to you?
- Do you have any questions?
- Do you understand the procedure?
- There are some risks involved with the procedure. Do you understand what they are?
- You could have some side-effects with this. Do you understand what they are?
- Do you understand what we hope to achieve with this procedure?
- Do you realise you can seek another opinion?
- Do you understand what other options there are?
- Are you still willing to proceed?
- Do you realise that you can withdraw from the procedure (or not) once it starts?

These are by no means exhaustive, but point to the importance of ensuring that there is full understanding of what the process is in the treatment or procedures being proposed.

In conclusion, it is worth noting that, in some cultures, it is not possible to ask an individual for consent, for the culture does not recognise the existence of autonomous individuals in the way they are recognised in Western culture. This means that consent is not just a matter for the individual, but may need to involve discussion with village elders or with the family. In seeking consent, healthcare professionals need to be aware of cultural differences that may affect how patients give consent, as well as issues of translation into another language. There is wisdom in some cultural practices that enshrine the need for broad consultation in relation to healthcare treatments and procedures, since this ensures that the individual's restoration to health is not just an individual problem, but one for the whole community to which they belong.

Reflective exercises

14.1 Is it ever justified not to ask patients to give informed consent? What if the treatment is too complex and an explanation affects the patient's mental state, and they become deeply depressed? What if the family members suggest, because it will be too traumatic, that it is wrong to tell their elderly father that he has only a few months to live if he does not agree to a particular treatment? Discuss.

14.2 Suppose the medical practitioner says that a person needs a biopsy, but states that that is all the patient needs to know. Is this enough for a patient to make an informed decision? How do we decide that enough information has been given? Discuss.

14.3 Is it okay if a health professional conversationally volunteers additional information about a procedure to a patient that is not on a consent form? What if the information confuses the patient? Discuss.

14.4 Suppose a colleague says that voluntary consent is a farce: the patient has to agree to the procedure or treatment if he wants to get better. Discuss some ways in which you could respond.

14.5 Can someone with a mental illness give voluntary informed consent? Discuss.

14.6 Is it ever justifiable to propose a treatment or procedure that does more harm than good? Discuss.

References

Aquinas, T. (1948). *Summa Theologica*, trans. Fathers of the Dominican Province. New York: Benziger Brothers.

Aristotle (1976). *Nichomachean ethics*, trans. J. A. K. Thomson, introduction and bibliography Jonathan Barnes (rev. ed. with notes and appendices H. Tredinnick). Harmondsworth: Penguin.

Australian and New Zealand College of Anaesthetists (2005). *Guidelines for consent to anaesthesia or sedation*. Retrieved 20 March 2014 from <http://www.safetyandquality.health.wa.gov.au/docs/consent/ANZCA_Guidelines_PS26_2005.pdf>.

Braun, A. R., Skene, L. & Merry, A. F. (2010). Informed consent for anaesthesia in Australia and New Zealand. *Anaesthesia and Intensive Care*, 38(5): 809–22.

Charlesworth, M. (1993). *Bioethics in a liberal society*. Cambridge: Cambridge University Press.

Corrigan, O. (2003). Empty ethics: The problem of informed consent. *Sociology of Health and Illness*, 25(3): 768–92.

Gillon, R. (1985). *Philosophical medical ethics*. Chichester: John Wiley and Sons.

Minors (Property and Contracts) Act 1970 (NSW).

Moran, C. & Lee, C. (2013). Selling genital cosmetic surgery to healthy women: A multimodal discourse analysis of Australian surgical websites. *Critical Discourse Studies*, 10(4): 373–91.

National Health and Medical Research Council (NHMRC) (2004). *General guidelines for medical practitioners on providing information to patients*. Canberra: Commonwealth of Australia.

O'Neill, O. (2004). *Autonomy and trust in bioethics*. Cambridge: Cambridge University Press.

Rendtorff, J. D. (2008). The limitations and accomplishments of autonomy as a basic principle in bioethics and biolaw, in D. N. Weisstub and G. D. Pintos (eds), *Autonomy and Human Rights in Health Care: An International Perspective*. New York: Springer.

World Medical Association (2006). *WMA International code of medical ethics*. Retrieved 20 March 2014 from <http://www.wma.net>.

15 The 'dead donor rule' and organ donation

Brigid McKenna

The transplantation of tissues and organs from deceased donors is well established in Australia, beginning with the first corneal transplant in 1941 and the first kidney transplants in the early 1960s (NHMRC, 2007). In 2013, a total of 391 deceased organ donors gave 1122 Australians a new chance in life after they received an organ transplant (Donate Life, 2014). Transplantation medicine is clearly one of the most dramatic success stories of modern medicine. It is, however, also one of the most ethically controversial, with significant personal, interpersonal and societal dimensions to consider. The practice of donation after death is a source of many of these controversies, especially when the demand for organs far exceeds their supply: around 1500 people are on Australian organ transplant waiting lists at any one time (Donate Life, 2014).

Transplantation medicine has always been guided by the primary ethical requirement that patients must be declared dead before any vital organs can be procured. However, the definition of death is not as straightforward as it once seemed. Whereas patients were once understood to be dead when they ceased to have evidence of circulation, respiration and brain functioning, with the loss of any one of these functions leading to the loss of the other two over a short period of time, the development of modern intensive-care medicine now allows the continuation of circulation and respiration in the absence of detectable brain function. This has made the question 'When is a person dead?' far more complicated (Truog & Robinson, 2003) and the ethical and legal requirements for organ donation far more controversial. This chapter critically examines the clinical and philosophical basis for the determination of death by neurological criteria ('brain death') and provides ethical analysis of emerging proposals for the ethical transplantation of vital organs.

Donation after death and the 'dead donor rule'

A primary ethical and legal principle guiding donation after death is often referred to as the 'dead donor rule' (DDR). The DDR states that donors must be dead before vital organs (for example, the heart, the entire liver, both kidneys) can be procured from their bodies. Additionally, the death of the patient must not be hastened, nor end-of-life care compromised in any way, to accommodate transplantation protocols (Pellegrino, 2008). To act otherwise would mean to intentionally cause the death of the donor for the purpose of transplantation. Glannon (2013: 192) explains the purpose of the DDR:

> The DDR is intended to ensure that severely compromised patients deemed potential donors are not killed for the sake of their organs. In this way, it protects transplant teams from the charge of murder and promotes public trust in the transplant system.

Yet, even if the DDR outlines the primary condition for the procurement of vital organs, its application will always rely upon consensus about what 'counts' as death. Australian state and territory laws have based their definitions of death on recommendations of the Australian Law Reform Commission (1977), where death is the:

- irreversible cessation of all function of the brain of the person, or
- irreversible cessation of circulation of blood in the body of the person.

The law does not specify the medical criteria that need to be met in order to verify that either of these conditions has been fulfilled. As is often the case, the law operates in conjunction with clinical guidelines, which further define and explain the terms and procedures necessary for the determination of death (Tonti-Filippini, 2012).

For instance, in Australia, the NHMRC guidelines (2007) explain that death determined by the irreversible loss of all brain function requires clinical confirmation of loss of brain-stem activity, the exclusion of factors that may temporarily have suppressed brain function and a causal link between the nature of the injury and loss of brain function. Further tests may be performed to confirm the absence of blood flow to the brain. In the alternative case of death determined by irreversible cessation of circulation, the guidelines refer to the need to ensure that resuscitative attempts are contraindicated on medical or legal grounds, and that there is no longer any possibility of auto-resuscitation.

Prior to 1970, vital organ procurement only occurred in the context of this second understanding of death – that is, after a donor's heart had irreversibly stopped beating. Indeed, it was not until 1968 that an ad hoc committee at the Harvard Medical School first published the report that formally instituted the concept of 'brain death' by defining death not only in terms of the irreversible cessation of circulation, but also as the irreversible cessation of all brain functions, including those of the brain stem. Guidelines were published for the management of patients with severe brain injuries who were comatose and showed no signs of recovery, but were being kept 'alive' by mechanical ventilation (Glannon, 2013).

Over time, however, the motives and conclusions of the Harvard Committee have become the subject of considerable criticism, despite the fact that the committee's work remains the basis for the substantive practice of donation after death around the world. One prominent critic, Alan Shewmon (2009), describes the reformulation of death in terms of brain function as a 'monumental socio-medico-legal revolution' in which the 'only rationale given by the committee for why the irreversible cessation of all brain functions should be equated with death was legal utility: it would free up beds in intensive care units and facilitate organ transplantation' (2009: 3). He also observes that this revolution rapidly unfolded without any consensus about official diagnostic criteria for the irreversible cessation of all brain function, or any philosophical rationale for why this should constitute death. Accordingly, today criticisms generally are raised in relation to three basic assumptions of the Harvard Committee: that patients who meet so-called 'Harvard criteria' in fact have lost all brain function; that patients who have lost all brain function are in fact dead; and that death is a necessary condition for removing vital organs (Fost, 2004).

'Testing' problems: Have patients who meet the 'Harvard criteria' lost all brain function?

There is no worldwide consensus on the medical criteria necessary for the diagnosis of 'brain death' (Wijdicks, 2002). Sometimes this is a result of different countries having different legal definitions of death by a neurological standard – for example, in contrast to the Australian definition outlined above, the United Kingdom defines death as *brain-stem* death, as evidenced by irreversible loss of the capacity for consciousness, combined with the irreversible loss of the capacity to breathe.

Furthermore, even where there is some consensus about what 'brain death' is, different countries may still use different criteria for determining the irreversible cessation of all brain function. In some countries (for example, France, Italy, Spain, Singapore), the required standard is that there must be evidence of zero blood volume transfer to the brain during angiography or Doppler ultrasound. In Australia, however, the Australian and New Zealand Intensive Care Society (ANZICS) states that testing for the irreversible loss of all brain function, and the consequent determination of brain death, only require unresponsive coma, the absence of brain-stem reflexes and the absence of respiratory centre function, in association with definite clinical or neuro-imaging evidence of acute brain pathology (such as traumatic brain injury, intracranial haemorrhage or hypoxic encephalopathy) consistent with the irreversible loss of neurological function. A test to show that there is an absence of blood supply to the brain is not required (Tonti-Filippini, 2012).

The significance of the existence of different diagnostic protocols is compounded further by the fact that it has been known for many years that some brain functions continue or linger on after traditional testing has shown irreversible cessation of all brain function. Persisting brain activity on electroencephalography, auditory and/or visual evoked potentials, as well as neuro-hormonal functioning via the hypothalamus or posterior pituitary (Halevy, 2001), demonstrate that the basic neurological criteria no longer suffice to measure the loss of all functions of the entire brain (Veatch, 2005).

Conceptual problems: Are patients who have lost all brain function in fact dead?

After the Harvard Committee report, more than 10 years passed before the 1981 President's Commission provided the first comprehensive philosophical rationale for equating the irreversible cessation of all brain function with death. This was based upon the view that 'the brain is the body's central integrator, without which the body necessarily and imminently literally "dis-integrates" and succumbs to asystole despite all technological interventions' (Shewmon, 2009: 4). By this account, the death of a person is understood to consist of the irreversible loss of bodily or 'somatic' integrative unity. Cells, individual organs and even bodily systems may remain 'alive', but the life of the person has ended (NHMRC, 2007).

Many religious views that see the person as an embodied spirit accept loss of integration as the departure of the soul. In general, however, there is widespread public confusion and scepticism about the concept of 'brain death'. People continue to describe 'brain-dead' patients being 'kept alive' by machines, or as 'dying' when the ventilator is withdrawn (Shewmon, 2009: 5). Others confuse 'brain death' with post-coma unresponsiveness or coma. Fost (2004: 251) observes that:

> For some, the standard is too high, as they believe a loved one has died long before the whole brain has ceased to function. For some, the standard is too low, as it is difficult to accept that a patient is dead when he appears to be sedated but otherwise normal, with good colour and all other organs func-tioning normally, and indistinguishable from many others in the intensive care unit whose status as 'alive' is not in question.

However, a more fundamental problem with the diagnosis of death by neuro-logical criteria is that, even if one were to *philosophically* equate death with the irreversible loss of the bodily integrative unity of the 'organism as a whole', it is highly questionable whether one could continue to *empirically* equate the death of the whole brain with the irreversible loss of the bodily integrative unity of the 'organism as a whole'. A significant body of evidence now demonstrates that many bodily integrative functions, such as homeostasis, elimination, energy balance, maintenance of body temperature, wound healing, fighting off infec-tions, development of a febrile response, cardiovascular and hormonal stress responses, and even the successful gestation of a foetus, sexual maturation and proportional growth, are *not* mediated by the brain. Each of these functions has been shown to occur in individuals diagnosed as 'brain dead' (Shewmon, 2001). Furthermore, documented cases of these people continuing to 'live', sometimes for years, further demonstrates that the body does not necessarily dis-integrate despite all technological support.

A decade and a half ago, Shewmon (1998) described the case of a TK, a young man who contracted meningitis at age four, for whom clinical testing showed no brain-stem function, evoked potentials showed no cortical or brain-stem responses, magnetic resonance angiogram showed no intracranial blood flow and an MRI scan revealed destruction of the entire brain, including the brain stem. Shewmon writes:

> Physicians suggested discontinuing support, but his mother would not hear of it. His early course was very rocky, but eventually he was transferred home, where he remains on a ventilator, assimilates food placed in his stomach by tube, urinates spontaneously, and requires little more than nursing care. While 'brain dead' he has grown, overcome infections, and healed wounds.
>
> ... TK has much to teach about the necessity of the brain for somatic integrative unity. There is no question that he became 'brain dead' at age four; neither is there any question that he is still alive at age nineteen. (1998: 136)

TK and others have demonstrated that, although the brain contributes more to bodily integrative unity than any other part of the body, life is not constituted solely by the brain. If the death of the whole brain is to be equated with death of the organism as a whole, it cannot be because of loss of somatic integrative unity (Shewmon, 2001). Indeed, perhaps 'brain death' is nothing more than a reliable criterion for establishing a prognosis of irreversibility (Rodríguez-Arias, Smith & Lazar, 2011).

What is 'death' and does it matter?

Death redefined

In the wake of this growing body of clinical research and philosophical inquiry, the majority position within the US President's Council on Bioethics (2008) rejected the loss of integration view as an explanation of brain death. In its place, the council proposed a new definition of death: 'the cessation of the fundamental vital work of a living organism – the work of self-preservation, achieved through the organism's need-driven commerce with the surrounding world' (2008: 60). According to this 'mode of being' view, it is acceptable to diagnose death if the living being is no longer receptive to stimuli, cannot act upon the world to obtain what it needs, and is not driven by basic felt needs. Clinically, this would mean that one could be satisfied that death had occurred on the basis of permanent loss of consciousness and spontaneous breathing, rather than the existing higher standard of loss of all functions of the brain. For example, the council's position admits that continued integration and some brain function, such as the hypo-thalamic pituitary axis in the mid-brain, could still be present in somebody who has been diagnosed as dead by the brain criteria (Tonti-Filippini, 2012).

This new 'definition' has received a mixed reception. Brugger (2013: 212) argues that even if the term 'fundamental work' of an organism is new and unique, its meaning as expressed in the three vital capacities necessary for life 'is essentially the "Harvard criteria" repackaged in the form of a philosophical justification'. The President's Council still leaves us, Brugger contends, with the questionable assumptions that patients who have suffered total brain failure have definitively ceased carrying out their vital work, therefore we can be morally certain that such patients are in fact dead. He concludes that the ongoing capacity for homeostasis, nutrition, wound healing and active immunity shown by some brain-dead bodies is an expression of the vital work of an organism – self-preservation – and enough to raise moral doubt that such patients are in fact dead.

In other critiques, Jones (2012) questions the arbitrary nature of the council's conclusions – specifically, why 'inner experience of need' should be chosen as essential to human life, given that it is not the most specific quality of human life, nor is it the most basic to biological life. He concludes that 'it is difficult to understand the rationale for the concept except as a device to defend the clinical status quo in the face of evidence of continuing somatic integration' (2012: 137). Shewmon (2009: 8–9) similarly criticises the mode of being view as a 'contortion of semantics' intended 'to save the neurological standard at all intellectual costs'. Tonti-Filippini (2012) raises the practical question of whether the medical understanding of death by the brain criterion will continue to be acceptable to many religious people now that the President's Council has rejected the explanation of 'brain death' in terms of loss of integration.

Higher brain death standard: 'As good as dead'

Another response to the problems associated with the determination of death by the brain criteria involves an even more radical amendment to the definition of death, which designates the loss of those brain functions that are responsible only for consciousness as the basis for pronouncing death.

Singer (1995) is one bioethicist who has popularised the view that a biologically living human being can be 'dead' on the grounds of loss/absence of personhood by virtue of permanent unconsciousness. For example, he says of individuals in an irreversible coma or a post-coma unresponsive ('vegetative') state, and anencephalic infants, that their organs can be removed because they have no prospect of regaining consciousness and continued life cannot benefit them. Veatch (2005) agrees, but with the qualification that both minimal somatic functions *and* minimal mental functions – what he describes as 'embodied consciousness' – are necessary for full moral standing to be present and a sufficient condition to be classified as 'alive'. By this account, a functional body without any capacity for mental function lacks the essential integration of body and mind, and should be considered a 'dead body' for public policy purposes such as homicide, inheritance, widowhood and organ procurement. Veatch also emphasises that the procurement of organs from these individuals should not be regarded as an 'exception' to the dead donor rule, but that such humans should be definitively classified as 'dead for purposes of social and public policy' on the basis that they have lost (or have never had) full moral standing.

This 'higher brain criterion', as it is often termed, was considered alongside the 'whole brain criterion' by the President's Commission (1981) and rejected: the permanent loss of what is essential to the nature of humans – consciousness – was found to be insufficient for the determination of death, as well as too impractical to assess with the certainly required for a statutory definition (Halevy, 2001). It was rejected again by the President's Council on Bioethics in 2008, which identified serious difficulties with the claim that something called 'death' can occur even as the body remains alive. These include the difficulty knowing that higher mental functions have been irreversibly lost, and the way in which this 'two deaths' position expands the concept of death beyond the core meaning it has had throughout human history, namely that human beings do not die as 'persons', but as members of the larger family of living beings and as animals in particular (p. 51). Further difficulties lie with the postulation that loss of personhood results in the coming to be of a new living entity, a kind of 'humanoid animal' that is human is some sense but that is not a human being (Jones, 2012). Founded upon a dualist conception of human life which abstracts personhood from human bodily life and, instead, identifies the 'person' with the mind or consciousness, arguably the use of a higher brain criteria is also highly elitist. As Fisher (2012: 224) argues:

> . . . even the severely cognitively impaired are living human beings: their life is their very reality as persons and as such remains a good, even if their life is not consciously enjoyed by them and however little it appeals to us. This is why we still care for persistently unresponsive people: such care ensures their participation in the goods of which they can still be subjects and maintains our bonds of interpersonal communion or solidarity with them. This also explains why we do not exploit or harm or bury alive such people or otherwise subject them to indignity.

Libertarian standard: 'Death by as many names'

Veatch (2005) proposes another response to the collapse of the concept of brain death, which seeks compromise in place of scientific and philosophical consensus. His position is based on the view that we live in a liberal society in which we should show tolerance and accommodation of the moral conclusions of different religious and philosophical traditions, so long as no one is significantly injured by doing so. Within a liberal society such as this, it might be preferable to adopt public policy that works on the basis of a default definition of death, with the provision that individuals should 'have the right to consciously reject the default position and opt for their own particular definition of death, that is, their own particular view about when full moral standing ends' (2005: 372).

There are, however, serious dangers involved with leaving the choice of the criteria for death to individual preference. It is precisely because of the expanding cultural and ethical pluralism of modern societies that public consensus about fundamental issues of human life and dignity is necessary for the common good. Without any stable criteria for death, it would be extremely difficult to maintain public trust in the integrity of organ transplantation after death, and consequently their involvement with organ donation programs. Pellegrino (2008: 113) cautions that:

> The need for organs, the desire to prolong life, and the potential 'good' to be done are forces difficult to control when death can be defined on one's own – or one's guardian's – terms. As experience has repeatedly shown, personal autonomy without moral constraint ends in divisive moral atomism. As difficult as the search for a common definition of death may be, that difficulty cannot justify abandoning the effort to establish a common definition.

Return to 'cardiac death': 'Be still my beating heart'

Another significant consequence of the conceptual and practical difficulties involved with brain death has been a renewed interest in the practice of 'donation after cardiac death' (DCD). This was, of course, how the first successful heart and liver transplants were carried out prior to the emergence of brain death. As well as supplanting the conceptual problems associated with brain death, DCD also creates the possibility of more organs being available for transplantation, give that many more people die through failure of the circulatory system.

'Controlled' DCD usually occurs in patients with catastrophic brain injuries who are ventilator dependent but do not meet the criteria for brain death. Mechanical ventilation is withdrawn in the operating theatre so that organs can be removed as soon as possible after the heart stops beating. To preserve organ quality, organs might be cooled in situ after death is declared, or catheters inserted prior to the declaration of death in order to maintain organ perfusion. The most significant variable, however, is the time required between loss of circulation and the declaration of death, which can be anywhere between 75 seconds and 10 minutes. 'Uncontrolled' DCD occurs after an unexpected cardiac arrest and unsuccessful attempts at resuscitation. Cardiac massage and ventilation are continued until the patient reaches hospital and a doctor rules out the possibility of the patient's recovery. Resuscitation is then stopped and death is declared following five further minutes of no circulatory function (Rodríguez-Arias, Smith & Lazar, 2011).

The critical question in relation to DCD protocols is precisely how long it takes for cessation of circulation to become 'irreversible' such that a valid declaration of death can occur and organ procurement can commence in accordance with the dead donor rule. How long, too, does it take for brain function – including the capacity to experience pain – to be irreversibly lost? Until consensus is reached about the answers to these questions, donors under DCD protocols could, like 'brain-dead' donors, also be alive at the time of vital organ procurement and at risk of suffering and intentional killing.

There are certainly other ethical issues in relation to DCD protocols, such as the legitimacy of undertaking interventions (e.g. inserting catheters before death to assist with organ preservation) that benefit potential recipients but offer no benefit, and possibly even some harm, to the donor; or the potential for medical care of dying patients to be influenced by the need to retrieve organs as soon after death. In the context of this discussion, however, the most pressing question is whether donation after cardiac death – like donation after the diagnosis of death by neurological criteria – routinely violates the dead donor rule and, if this is the case, where this leaves the practical and ethical basis for the donation of vital organs after death.

Abandon the dead donor rule: 'Why wait for death?'

At least in the literature, the view that the current practice of vital organ donation routinely violates the DDR has led to repeated calls for the rule to be abandoned and for the adoption of an alternative basis for the ethical procurement of vital organs (Glannon, 2013; Miller, Truog & Brock, 2010; Rodríguez-Arias, Smith & Lazar, 2011; Truog & Robinson, 2003; Wilkinson & Savulescu, 2012).

Miller, Truog and Brock (2010) argue that the fundamental norm that doctors must not intentionally kill patients is *not* absolute, given that, in their view, the widely accepted practice of stopping life-sustaining treatment is itself an act of medical killing, and not merely allowing a patient to die. When a patient dies under such circumstances, the only difference between an act of homicide and the legitimate withdrawal of treatment is whether the patient has consented to the withdrawal of treatment. With this assumption in the background, they argue:

> Given that it is ethical to cause death by withdrawing life-sustaining treatment, it cannot be presumed that it is necessarily unethical to procure vital organs from living patients prior to withdrawing treatment. Indeed, it is the consent of the patient or surrogate in each case that underlies the fundamental ethical justification of each practice. (2010: 305)

Miller, Truog and Brock reject the suggestion that procuring vital organs from living patients could be exploitative by insisting upon valid consent and limiting vital organ donation to patients with prior justified plans to withdraw life-sustaining treatment, made independently of any decision about organ donation. The importance of this, they argue, is that: 'no patient would die as a result of organ donation who would not otherwise soon die from withdrawing treatment. In that sense, no person is being killed in order to save the life of another' (2010: 306).

Wilkinson and Savulescu (2010) rely upon similar arguments to advance a proposal for 'organ donation euthanasia' (ODE). According to their utilitarian calculus, ODE promises less suffering and a greater range and number of viable organs, and provides (consenting) individuals with the greatest possible chance of donating their organs. Wilkinson and Savulescu concede that ODE would be a form of direct killing or 'euthanasia', and in direct conflict with the DDR and the injunction against medical killing. Yet, so long as patients give consent for ODE, they reject the widely held view that patients will be morally harmed or have their rights violated if they are actively killed, any more than if they consented to die as a result of treatment withdrawal.

Such views are, however, a radical departure from the traditional understanding of the role of intention in ethical decision-making to withhold or withdraw life-sustaining treatment. There is often a critical ethical difference between 'killing' and 'letting die', depending upon whether death is directly intended or merely foreseen as a side-effect, even if the physical acts or omissions sometimes appear outwardly identical. The absolute prohibition of medical killing does not preclude the withdrawal of life-sustaining treatment where such treatment is withdrawn because it is medically futile or overly burdensome. Unlike the deliberate procurement of vital organs from a living patient, withdrawing treatment under these circumstances is not intentional killing; it simply respects the patient's right to inviolability and allows them to die from natural causes.

Opponents of the dead donor rule also argue that, even if they are not biologically dead, because patients diagnosed with brain death are in an irreversible coma, they have ceased to exist as a person and are *unable to be harmed* or wronged by extracting vital organs prior to stopping life-sustaining treatment. (Miller, Truog & Brock, 2010; Wilkinson & Savulescu, 2012). Somewhat ironically, Glannon (2013: 201) suggests that adherence to the DDR might in fact cause harm:

> Waiting until all neurological and circulatory functions have permanently ceased before removing organs may cause nonexperiential harm for the potential donor by causing ischemia, rendering his or her organs nonviable for transplantation. It could also harm potential transplant recipients by defeating their interest in receiving a transplant.

Again, however, this notion of 'harm' relies upon the highly contested view that permanently unconscious patients are non-persons. The President's Council on Bioethics (2008: 71) concluded that it would be both 'conceptually suspect and practically dangerous' to expect that the principle of non-maleficence – of 'do no harm' – could provide sufficient ethical safeguards for procuring organs from the living:

> What exactly does 'harm' mean in this context, and how do we know who is beyond harm? Might there be a temptation to interpret the class of 'patients who can still be harmed' more and more narrowly in order to increase the number of donation eligible human beings? (2008: 71)

Clearly, if the DDR were to be abandoned, it would be difficult to justify why vital organ donation should be limited to settings involving the withdrawal of life-sustaining treatment. In fact, Miller, Truog and Brock (2010) concede that they would not regard a healthy person of sound mind making a self-sacrificing organ donation to save the life of a loved one as unethical *per se*. They merely observe that it would be exceedingly rare that any competent clinical team would be prepared to comply with such a plan. If consent were to become the primary determinant of ethical practice, in principle as well as in practice, it would be difficult to refuse a voluntary and rational request to donate vital organs, even where the primary motivation was not altruism, but suicide.

Ultimately, the moral integrity of live vital organ donation or 'organ donation euthanasia' cannot be derived from the expression of self-determination (potential organ donors) and the relief of suffering for others (potential organ recipients). There are many actions that remain morally wrong, even if they are freely and intelligently chosen, and capable of max-imising good outcomes. Fisher (2012: 222) writes, somewhat confrontingly, that:

> People, especially weak people, who respond to the invitation of authoritative others to renounce their inviolability, are not exercising autonomy. Homicidal acts or omissions do not become right simply by becoming policies or by getting the victims to sign their own death warrants.

Except for a handful of jurisdictions around the world, healthcare ethics, the law and society continue to hold that the direct killing of another individual – even with that individual's consent – is morally wrong. It deprives people of the basic good of human life, contravenes the right not to be killed, undermines the value of respect for human life, violates trust and, in this instance, places healthcare professionals at the service of death rather than life. Allowing doctors to kill their patients would fundamentally distort the doctor–patient relationship and violate both the goals of medicine and a basic societal norm:

> Even if an individual is 'brain dead', killing him for the good of others cannot be justified. Crossing that line is dangerous for patients, who are some of the weakest members of society and dependent upon its protection. (Potts & Evans, 2005: 408)

The DDR upholds the Kantian categorical imperative to treat living human beings as an end in themselves, and not merely as a means to another human being's ends – a principle that has been fundamental to the ethics of both biomedical research and clinical medicine at least since the promulgation of the

Nuremberg Code in 1947 (President's Council on Bioethics, 2008). For many people, the practice of organ transplantation is ethically defensible precisely because only those who are already dead are eligible to become donors. Abandoning the DDR would generate fear and undermine the more general acceptance of, and confidence in, organ donation and transplantation.

Conclusion

At least for the moment, there remain serious practical and philosophical problems with the determination of death by neurological criteria. This is particularly troubling, given that organ donation after death is still largely only performed in cases where a patient is declared 'brain dead' in an intensive-care setting. One of the most influential clinicians and thinkers in this area, Professor Alan Shewmon, observes (2009: 6) that:

> 'Brain death as death' began as a utilitarian legislative decree and has remained a conclusion in search of a justification ever since: a conclusion clung to at all costs for the sake of the transplantation enterprise that quickly came to depend on it.

Given the weight of clinical and philosophical opposition to the concept, perhaps the time has come to finally abandon the 'conclusion' and explore new ethical premises for donation after death. The expansion of a properly regulated practice of donation after cardiac death might provide an acceptable alternative – although, as we have briefly seen, this will require some serious ethical issues to be addressed. There is certainly more merit to this venture than there is to extreme proposals to either declare living patients dead or abandon the requirement that patients are in fact dead before procuring organs for transplantation. The integrity of transplantation medicine will stand or fall with the fate of the 'dead donor rule'.

Reflective exercises

15.1 A primary ethical and legal principle guiding donation after death is often referred to as the 'dead donor rule' (DDR). What is the main clinical criterion for this principle? Compare the clinical criterion to donation after cardiac death (DCD). Are there any complexities in this comparison that could result in the health professional facing an ethical dilemma in clinical practice?

15.2 What are the main clinical testing processes in the Harvard Committee criteria to determine brain death? Do you think Alan Shewmon's criticism of the Harvard Committee criteria for brain-death testing is justifiable?

15.3 The United Kingdom defines death as brain-stem death, which is evidenced by irreversible loss of the capacity for consciousness, combined with the irreversible loss of the capacity to breathe. This differs from the Australian legal and clinical definition of death. What are the ethical, clinical and social implications of the UK definition for brain-death determination required for organ donation?

15.4 Review the Australian and New Zealand Intensive Care Society (ANZICS) statement on brain death and organ donation at <http://www.anzics.com.au>. What is ANZIC's definition on brain death? What are the clinical pre-condition criteria to undertake brain death testing and why are these criteria required?

15.5 In recent years, the apnoea test that may be part of the clinical testing for brain death has come under some scrutiny, with some medical professionals questioning whether eliciting hypercapnoeia is ethical. Do you think that this criticism is justifiable?

15.6 Are human beings who have lost the capacity for consciousness no longer members of the human species? Is sixteenth-century French philosopher Rene Descartes' suggestion that 'I think, therefore I am' essentially true? Discuss by highlighting the higher brain criterion for brain death in your argument.

15.7 'The definition of brain death has collapsed.' Discuss this statement with reference to the historical origins, philosophical basis and challenges to the conventional concept of 'brain death'. What ethical issues are raised by challenges to the concept of brain death?

15.8 What are the key clinical features of the US President's Council on Bioethics' 'mode of being' view? What are the ethical, legal and social implications for this diagnosis in the clinical setting, and in relation to organ donation?

References

Australian Government (2014). Organ and Tissue Authority. *Donation facts and statistics*. Retrieved 13 April 2014 from <http://temp.donatelife.gov. au/media/docs/The_Authority/ Accountability_and_Reporting/ Donation_Facts_and_Statistics_-_ January_2014.pdf>.

Australian Law Reform Commission (1977). *ALRC 7. Report of the Law Reform Commission on Human Tissue Transplants*. Canberra: Australian Government Publishing Service.

Brugger, C. (2013). Alan Shewmon and the PCBE's White Paper on brain death: Are brain-dead patients dead? *Journal of Medicine and Philosophy*, 38(2): 205–18.

Donate Life (2014). Website. Retrieved 20 September 2014 from <http://www.donatelife.gov.au>.

Fisher, A. (2012). *Catholic bioethics for a new millennium*. New York: Cambridge University Press.

Fost, N. (2004). Reconsidering the dead donor rule: Is it important that organ donors be dead? *Kennedy Institute of Ethics Journal*, 14(3): 249–60.

Glannon, W. (2013). The moral insignificance of death in organ donation. *Cambridge Quarterly of Healthcare Ethics*, 22: 192–202.

Halevy, A. (2001). Beyond brain death? *Journal of Medicine and Philosophy*, 26(5): 493–501.

Jones, D. A. (2012). Loss of faith in brain death: Catholic controversy over the determination of death by neurological criteria. *Clinical Ethics*, 7(3): 133–41.

Miller, F., Truog, R. & Brock, D. (2010). The dead donor rule: Can it withstand critical scrutiny? *Journal of Medicine and Philosophy*, 35: 299–312.

National Health and Medical Research Council (NHMRC) (2007). *Organ and tissue donation after death, for transplantation*. Canberra: Australian Government Publishing Service.

Pellegrino, E. (2008). *Personal statement. Controversies in the determination of death: A white paper*. Washington, DC: President's Council on Bioethics.

Potts, M. & Evans, D. W. (2005). Does it matter that organ donors are not dead? Ethical and policy implications. *Journal of Medical Ethics*, 31: 406–9.

President's Commission for the Study of Ethical Problems in Medicine and Biomedical and Behavioral Research (1981). *Defining death: Medical, legal and ethical issues in the determination of death*. Washington, DC: Government Printing Office.

President's Council on Bioethics (2008). *Controversies in the determination of death: A white paper*. Washington, DC: President's Council on Bioethics. Retrieved 20 April 2014 from <https://bioethicsarchive.georgetown.edu/pcbe/reports/death>.

Rodríguez-Arias, D., Smith, M.J & Lazar, N. M. (2011). Donation after circulatory death: Burying the dead donor rule. *The American Journal of Bioethics*, 11(8): 36–43.

Shewmon, D. A. (1998). 'Brainstem death,' 'brain death' and death: A critical re-evaluation of the purported equivalence. *Issues in Law & Medicine*, 14(2): 125–45.

—— (2001). The brain and somatic integration: insights into the standard biological rationale for equating 'brain death' with death.

Journal of Medicine and Philosophy, 26: 457–78.

—— (2009). Brain death: Can it be resuscitated? *Issues in Law & Medicine*, 25(1): 3–14.

Singer, P. (1995). *Rethinking life and death*. Oxford: Oxford University Press.

Tonti-Filippini, N. (2009). Has the definition of death collapsed? *Bioethics Research Notes*, 21(4): 79–82.

—— (2012) Religious and secular death: A parting of the ways. *Bioethics*, 26 (8): 410–21.

Truog, R. & Robinson, W. (2003). Role of brain death and the dead-donor rule in the ethics of organ transplantation. *Critical Care Medicine*, 31(9): 2391–6.

Veatch, R. M. (2005). The death of whole-brain death: The plague of the disaggregators, somaticists, and mentalists. *Journal of Medicine and Philosophy*, 30(4): 353–78.

Wijdicks, E. F. M. (2002). Brain death worldwide: Accepted fact but no global consensus in diagnostic criteria. *Neurology*, 58(20): 20–5.

Wilkinson, D. & Savulescu, J. (2012). Should we allow organ donation euthanasia? Alternatives for maximizing the number and quality of organs for transplantation. *Bioethics*, 26(1): 32–48.

16 Just care at the end of life

Bernadette Tobin

Providing good care – medical and nursing – to people whose lives are drawing to an end continues to pose challenges for Australians. The challenges include both practical and ethical ones. Among the practical issues are those to do with how to ensure access to good end-of-life care – in particular, palliative care – to everyone to whom it is owed. Among the ethical concerns are questions to do with how best to understand *what* is *owed* to *whom*. This discussion will focus on the ethical issues. Although the writer of the Hippocratic Oath insists that it is part of a doctor's duty to keep his patients free from injustices they can do to *themselves*, justice is generally understood to be what is owed to *others*. The idea of what is owed to others can be understood in a range of ways – from the relatively specific idea of fulfilling responsibilities defined by prior undertakings to the relatively inclusive idea of acting uprightly in *any* actions that have a bearing on others. In the former sense, justice is often referred to as 'fairness', and in the latter sense it is often a label for the whole of virtue. In the first section of this chapter, I outline four ways in which justice as what is owed to others is understood: a 'utilitarian' understanding, a 'libertarian' understanding, an 'egalitarian' understanding and a 'pluralist' understanding.[1] I will briefly indicate what I take to be the strengths and weaknesses of each approach, explaining why I think the pluralist view is the most reasonable. I will also touch on an independent but related issue: how each approach tends to view the other – the person to whom justice is owed. In the second section, I will assume a 'pluralist' understanding of justice, and spell out one of its implications for the treatment and care of people at the end of their lives so that they have genuine choices in treatment and forms of care.

Four approaches to justice in the distribution of healthcare resources

Since no society can afford to provide all the healthcare that its citizens need, let alone want, the community should allocate it justly (Tobin, 2002). There are four different ways in which what constitutes justice in the allocation of health-care resources might be understood. There is overlap between them and much variety of approach within each. So what follows is a general outline of the key ideas that characterise each, followed by a brief indication of the strengths and weaknesses of the approach.

A 'utilitarian' approach: Whatever brings about utility

According to utilitarianism, justice is not an independent moral principle. Rather, it is a principle dependent on and governed by the sole principle of morality: the principle of utility. Justice names that most paramount and stringent form of obligation created by the principle of utility. The principle of utility says: identify the foreseeable benefits and the foreseeable losses of a proposal or state of affairs, calculate the net sum (or utility) of benefits minus losses and adopt the state of affairs that will bring about the greatest good for the greatest number – that will 'maximise' utility. Justice consists in the result of that calculation. A state of affairs is just if it represents the greatest good for the greatest number and unjust if it fails to represent that result.

In healthcare, quality-of-life measures and social contribution measures are used to determine utility (Singer, 2009). Although different utilitarians advocate different specific policies, they favour a number of things:

- prevention rather than cure, the cheaper rather than the more expensive, the short term rather than the long term
- priority to the young ahead of the old
- preference to be given to those likely to receive greater benefit rather than lesser benefit
- the lowest priority given to healthcare for the terminally ill, dying, elderly, chronically sick or incapacitated, handicapped or permanently unconscious (Fisher, 1994).

Peter Singer (1979) has used utilitarianism to argue that the affluent have obligations to the poor – particularly to the poor who live in far-away places. He has also used it to reveal what is wrong with cultural relativism in ethics (which is relevant to thinking about our obligations to the very young and the very old), and to underline the importance of efficiency and effectiveness in healthcare. So a utilitarian emphasis on 'outcomes' has its merits. That said, utilitarianism captures only a part of what is true in morality. Consequences ('outcomes') matter, but they are not the only thing that matters. Utilitarianism pays little attention to individual rights and duties, and thus to the moral significance of particular relationships. In its insistence on 'maximising' good consequences, it may not only ask too much of us but also may invite us to consider doing evil for the sake of good. When it is combined with a contemporary account of personhood – one that derives from John Locke – utilitarianism threatens to undermine the authentic goal of healthcare.

An 'egalitarian' approach: An equal distribution of goods and services

According to egalitarianism, justice is essentially equality or, following the most influential of contemporary egalitarians, fairness. Unlike utilitarians (who think that ultimately there is only one moral principle, utility), egalitarians treat justice as one among a plurality of moral principles, of which benevolence (say) is another.

John Rawls (1971), the best-known exponent of contemporary egalitarianism, says that principles of justice can be derived from what people would choose if they were forced to be impartial – if (behind a 'veil of ignorance') they had to choose principles on which to base a social structure that would satisfy them wherever they turned out to be located in that society. He argues that, behind such a veil of ignorance, people would choose two principles: first, each person would have the most extensive system of basic liberties compatible with similar liberties for all; and second, social and economic inequalities would be arranged so that they were to the greatest benefit of the least advantaged and open to all under conditions of fair equality of opportunity. In brief, justice consists in fair equality of opportunity.

Rawls did not apply his theory to the allocation of healthcare. Though its application to healthcare is a matter of some debate, Rawls-inspired approaches to healthcare distribution, such as that of Norman Daniels (2008), insist that fairness requires that everyone, regardless of wealth or social status, should have access to the basic healthcare resources that are needed to ensure that each person enjoys an equal opportunity with everyone else to lead a good life. What is a 'good life'? Rawls argues that the state must be neutral about that. Its arrangements for healthcare, education and so on must provide the maximum scope for each person to determine their own personal values and life-plans.

This 'thin theory of the good' recognises only those 'primary goods' that people need to pursue their particular plans and projects, together with a few principles of justice-as-fairness. On this account, healthcare ought to be understood as care that provides or restores opportunities in life to those whose opportunities are limited by illness. Healthcare needs are whatever is necessary to achieve, restore and maintain equality of opportunities. Better services, such as private hospital rooms and cosmetic but optional dental work, should be available for purchase at personal expense by those who have the money and the desire to do so. But everyone's basic health needs should be met at a level that is adequate for equality of opportunity. On Rawls' and Daniels' view, we can talk of a right to a 'decent minimum' of healthcare – enough to ensure equality of opportunity. Justice requires that the society provides this to all its citizens.

In my view, egalitarianism marks an advance on utilitarianism in that it recognises that there is an irreducible plurality of moral values: utility is one value, equality is another, benevolence a third, and so on. Rawls' theory suggests an approach to justice that, while respecting the individuality of person and the diversity of the conditions in which they flourish, attempts to set out a reasoned basis for a harmonious life between individuals. It rightly claims that 'need' is the criterion for the proper distribution of healthcare. And it rightly reminds us of what is owed, as a matter of social justice or fairness, to the poor and disadvantaged. On the other hand, Fisher and Gormally (2001) point to a range of problems it generates. For instance, how can the state determine what level of healthcare is needed for equality of opportunity if it is neutral about what constitutes the good life that each is to have an equal opportunity to live? And is equality of opportunity the only value we seek and express in healthcare? Is not solidarity with those who suffer as a result of illness another value we seek and express in our provision of healthcare?

A 'libertarian' approach: Lack of restraints on individual liberty

Rawls' theory of justice as fairness provides a useful backdrop against which to understand a third, libertarian, approach to justice. Robert Nozick's (1968: ix) claim that 'individuals have rights, and there are things no person or group may do to them without violating their rights' is a famous modern expression of a libertarian approach to justice. According to libertarianism, it is not the role of the state to impose any pattern of distribution of benefits and burdens on its members, since that will violate the rights of individuals. The state should not violate the rights of individuals: to life, to liberty, to property and so on. Individuals are entitled to exercise their rights free of interference from others, as long as they do not thereby interfere with the similar rights of others. The sole function of the state is to protect citizens against unjust interference – for example, by violence, theft, fraud or the non-fulfilment of contracts. It is not the business of the state to distribute benefits and burdens such as healthcare, since that will violate the rights of individuals. The role of the state is simply the limited one of a 'night watchman'.

According to libertarianism, it is a matter for individuals how much they choose to spend on healthcare. It is up to individuals to decide what healthcare (or healthcare insurance) to obtain, and which doctors or hospitals to obtain it from. According to libertarianism, it is up to healthcare professionals to decide to whom they will provide healthcare, when they will provide it, how they will provide it and how much they will charge for it. Therefore, the only just 'system' for the allocation of healthcare resources is the operation of the free market. Libertarians thus treat autonomy – both of the patient and of the healthcare professional – as the central ethical notion in healthcare. Individuals must be encouraged to take responsibility for their own health (Dworkin, 1981). They should not look to others to bail them out, nor should others be ready to do this: even well-meaning charity may have the side-effect of discouraging people from taking responsibility for themselves. Of course, it is unfortunate if some cannot pay for their own healthcare (or healthcare insurance), but it is not unfair that this is so. And even if it is unfortunate if a doctor does not wish to treat certain categories of people – the very poor, the homeless, people of a certain skin colour, people of a certain ethnic background – it is nonetheless not unfair. For the doctor–patient relationship should be understood as a relationship between two autonomous, contracting individuals. Healthcare workers are obliged to provide only the healthcare that is in keeping with their own prior undertakings or present choices. They may legitimately decide for themselves what distribution standards to apply to their own practices: profit maximisation through an 'ability to pay' criterion, personal satisfaction through a 'preferred group criterion' or some more altruistic criterion.

Applying Nozick's libertarianism to healthcare, Engelhardt (1986: 336) argues that 'a basic human right to the delivery of healthcare, even to the delivery of a decent minimum of healthcare, does not exist'. Nor, he adds, does anyone have a responsibility to provide it for others. A taxation system that supports the provision of healthcare for everyone actually perverts justice in that it places unreasonable restraints on individual liberty. Organs, babies, the use of women's wombs may all be transferred for money by individuals in a free market. Though a libertarian will not be opposed to any mode of healthcare distribution that has been freely chosen by a group, they will generally prefer a system in which healthcare insurance is privately and voluntarily purchased by individual initiative.

Libertarians are right to insist that healthcare is not (or is not entirely) a common resource that is to be distributed according to some formula. Those who work in healthcare are not merely 'resources' to be distributed according to someone else's interests or grand plan. There is also something right in libertarianism's emphasis on the responsibility of the individual to look after their own life and health, together with that of dependants. But libertarianism takes both of these ideas too far. Healthcare workers do not 'own' their labours. Their knowledge, skill and judgement are not purely of their own creation, even though they have used their own free will and individual motivation in their cultivation. Healthcare workers are educated to a significant degree at the public expense – usually in public institutions – and the knowledge they receive is a social product not of their own making. In addition, without a high level of social collaboration, there would be no sophisticated hospitals and medical schools. So too much emphasis on the idea that it is the responsibility of each individual to preserve and maintain their own health may overlook the importance of the fact that many things that influence health – poverty, social class, ignorance and genetic predisposition, to name just a few – lie beyond the scope of individual responsibility.

A 'pluralist' approach: Do unto others what you would have them do unto you

Utility, equality, liberty, solidarity – indeed, life and health – are all 'common' goods, which means they are good for everyone, regardless of differences between societies, cultures or individual preferences. A pluralist approach (Buckle, 1991) starts from this plurality of irreducible goods, and understands justice to be the favouring and fostering of the plurality of common goods of the community. Aristotle (1976) said that when men are friends they have no need of justice – the truest form of justice is a friendly quality. He meant that, in a decent ('just') society, individuals value not only their own 'flourishing' (their own life and health and knowledge and leisure), but also the flourishing of others. John Finnis (1980: viii) puts it this way: 'Few will flourish and no one will flourish securely unless there is effective collaboration between members of a community and co-ordination of their resources and enterprises.' Common enterprises are not ends in themselves, but rather means of assistance to individuals. So one part of justice requires distributing things that are essentially common, but that must be appropriated to individuals if they are to serve the common good: resources, opportunities, profits and advantages, roles and offices, responsibilities, taxes and burdens. Given that the objective of justice is the common good, and consequently the flourishing of all members of the community, a distribution is just if it is a reasonable solution to the problem of allocating the things that are essentially common but that need – for the sake of the common good – to be appropriated to individuals. Proportionality rather than equality is the key to recognising the demands of distributive justice. Inequalities of wealth are not unjust *per se*. What is unjust is the failure of the affluent to redistribute that part of their wealth that could be better used by others for obtaining and enjoying basic goods in *their* lives.

Anthony Fisher (1994) has worked out the details of such a 'pluralist' approach to the allocation of healthcare (he calls it a 'neo-Aristotelian' approach). Starting from the idea that healthcare truly is – at least in some regards – an allocable resource, he argues that it ought to be distributed according to what he calls the 'Golden Rule of healthcare'. This Golden Rule sets a two-part test of any allocation:

> Would I think that a healthcare budget and principles of allocation were fair if I (or someone I loved) were in healthcare need, especially if I were one of those excluded from provision or were among the weakest in the community, i.e. sick with a chronic, disabling and expensive ailment, poor, illiterate, etc? Would I think them fair were I (or someone I loved) a healthcare worker, a healthcare planner, a taxpayer and/or an insurer? (1994: 135; Fisher & Gormally, 2001: 98)

Applying this two-part test, Fisher argues that the primary basis for healthcare distribution is simply healthcare *need*, where satisfaction of that need is compatible with the fulfilment of similar or more important needs of other members of that community. The concept of need here is not 'capacity to benefit', nor 'what is required for self-determination', but more generally (along with food, water, clothing, shelter, exercise, freedom, safety, rest and family) what is required for participation in the goods of human life and health. There is thus a certain necessary indeterminacy in the concept of healthcare *need*. Customs, expectations, standards of living and current technology all influence people's perception of their needs. That said, interventions that are not oriented to human life and health, but that (like many forms of cosmetic surgery) serve some other goal, are not responses to genuine healthcare needs. For, as Hippocrates said, the specific goal of healthcare is 'the good of the *sick person*'.

Pluralist approaches do not generate absolutely general rules of healthcare distribution. For this reason, some healthcare administrators are impatient about a pluralist approach to justice in the allocation of healthcare resources. No doubt because they have to make very difficult and complex distributive decisions, according to which the needs of some patients and categories of patient inevitably must take priority over the needs of other patients and categories of patients, healthcare administrators are sometimes attracted by the distributive simplicity promised by a 'quality-adjusted life year' algorithm or a 'disability-adjusted life year' algorithm. To my mind, however, a pluralist approach is the most reasonable of the four approaches to justice. Like the utilitarian approach, it insists on the value of impartiality, and the importance of efficiency and efficacy. Like the egalitarian approach, it insists on what is owed – as a matter of justice – by the relatively affluent to the relatively poor and vulnerable. Like the libertarian approach, it recognises the moral importance of respect for personal decision-making. But, unlike any of them, it does not over-simplify things, for it recognises that there is a plurality of social goods at stake in the just distribution of healthcare. And, at least in its Christian expression, it highlights the great ideal of human solidarity. What the rich person owes to the poor, the healthy person to the sick, the independent person to the dependent, and so on, is not merely a matter of fairness: it is also a matter of solidarity with, and compassion for, that other person.

Who counts as 'the other'?

Utilitarianism has no official answer to this question, except to insist on impartiality in the calculation of benefits and burdens. In practice, however, the most influential utilitarians in the field of bioethics tend to exclude certain categories of human beings from counting as persons to whom we have obligations in justice. The Australian utilitarian philosopher Peter Singer combines his utilitarianism with John Locke's view about who counts as 'the other'. John Locke (1975: 335) defined a person as a 'thinking intelligent being that has reason and reflection and can consider itself as itself, the same thinking being, in different times and places'. Singer (1994) argues both that certain categories of human beings – newly born infants, the permanently comatose, the cognitively compromised – are not persons, and that certain groups of non-humans – gorillas, chimpanzees, the higher apes – might turn out to be persons.

Nor does egalitarianism have an official view of who counts as the other. Rawls tends to assume that individuals are to be understood as conscious and free moral agents who devise, revise and seek to achieve their own conceptions of the good. This has implications for those human beings who are not at a particular time, or may never be, competent moral agents. As Fisher (1994) points out, it at least invites a distributive preference in favour of those who are, or will be, capable of exercising moral agency.

Nor does libertarianism have an official view of who counts as the other. However, Engelhardt combines his version of libertarianism with a commit-ment not only to a Lockean notion of personhood, but also to the idea that it is only 'persons' who really matter: 'Persons, not humans, are special . . . obliga-tions of respect or beneficence vary according to the moral status of the entities involved' (1986: 104–5). Indeed, the centrality of autonomy in Nozick's theory would seem to support a 'consciousness criterion' in the allocation of healthcare resources. Those who can exercise moral agency ought to be preferred to those who cannot. And, of course, those who bring ill-health on themselves certainly ought not to be rescued by the state, for in using taxes for this purpose, the state will inevitably violate the rights of others.

Nor, finally, does pluralism have an official view on this matter. Certainly Aristotle seemed to think that what is owed as a matter of justice is owed *only* to male members of one's political community. However, today a vibrant expres-sion of a pluralist view is found in Catholic Christianity's valuing of human life itself, according to which not only is every human being to be treated as one's neighbour, but there is also a special obligation of solidarity with the poor and the vulnerable. A 'preferential option' for the poor supports a strong commit-ment to the care of individuals who are very young or very old, disabled or frail, sick or cognitively impaired – and indeed to those who may well have con-tributed to their own ill-health. This particular expression of a pluralist view of ethics rejects as unjust the idea that only those who possess 'personhood' are the proper recipients of healthcare (Williams, 1985). Nor is the provision of healthcare to the poor only an expression of justice; it also expresses compassion and fellow-feeling for those who suffer, encouragement and support for those who are disabled, gratitude to those who have benefited one, solidarity with those who approach death, love and friendship for those who are one's dependants, and so on. For, as we have seen, it insists that a healthcare system is to be evaluated against standards set by a plurality of social goods.

It can be seen that there are commonalities and overlaps between utilitarian, egalitarian, libertarian and pluralist conceptions of justice in the allocation of healthcare resources – in particular to those who are at the end of their lives. That said, each approach provides a distinctive starting point for thinking about what justice requires at the end of life. It is that specific subject that is addressed in what follows.

What justice requires at the end of life

Sudden death is now rare. Even death after a 'terminal illness' happens mostly to young people. Most Australians will die at an old age, after gradual organ failure or as a result of the gradual dwindling of their capacities. Healthcare successes of the last half-century mean that, for many, death will come after people have lost the capacity to talk to their healthcare professional and to those who care for them about what they would want by way of medical treatment. In an affluent country like Australia, where virtually everyone has access to sophisticated healthcare treatment, this will often be problematic. Most who die in hospital will do so after a decision has been made *not* to do something. The crucial decision-making imposes great burdens, not only on the healthcare professionals (trained to save lives!), but also on the relatives who are consulted. It is so stressful that families are sometimes unable to agree among themselves as to what it is best to do. In addition, increasing numbers of Australians have no relatives to contribute to the decision-making process. How, then, can the elderly have genuine choices about their treatment and care at the end of life? Once again, the challenges are both practical and ethical. In what follows, I shall set out some key ethical ideas that, at home in a pluralist conception of justice in the distribution of healthcare resources, ought to inform policies for the treatment and care of people who are approaching the end of their lives. The key idea will be that their treatment and care should be oriented 'to the good of the sick person', and should also reflect that person's judgements about how they wish to live the last part of their life. Since the emphasis will be on people who are no longer able to make decisions about their own treatment and care, the discussion can usefully be read as a discussion about the moral significance of 'advance-care planning'.

At its best, advance-care planning is planning for the future to ensure that the proper goals of healthcare treatment inform the care of people who become unable to make decisions about their own treatment, and that the means used to seek those goals reflect the judgements (the 'choices') of the patient. Such planning is an extension of the idea, found in the Judeo-Christian expressions of the pluralist tradition, of the legitimacy of an individual's forgoing of 'extraordinary' means of treatment. As Sulmasy (2008) points out, it springs from key principles found in the pluralist tradition: the dignity of the human person, the *prima facie* duty to preserve life, the fact of finitude and the diversity of the human. (The term 'extraordinary' simply means 'optional'.)

What goals and means are proper to healthcare? The goals of healthcare include promoting health and preventing disease; saving life, curing illness and slowing the progress of a disease; relieving suffering and disability; and caring for people when they are sick, disabled, frail or elderly (Catholic Health Australia, 2001). The means used to pursue those goals should be therapeutic ones – that is, they should be oriented to the health of the patient. Healthcare professionals should therefore have a clear understanding of the purpose for which they propose an intervention (for example, to provide diagnostic or prognostic information; to save a life; to improve or maintain the patient's health by curing an illness or slowing the course of an illness or by stabilising a patient in a reasonably satisfactory condition; to relieve pain or other symptoms of illness; to nourish and sustain a patient). And they should endeavour to ensure that patients – and their families – clearly understand the purpose for which an intervention is proposed. Treatments that are futile (that is, they will not work: they will not cure the patient; they will not make a significant contribution to improvement in the patient's condition; they will not appreciably forestall an imminent death) or overly burdensome (that is, the benefits hoped for – whether physical, psychological, social, economic, moral or spiritual – do not justify the foreseeable burdens imposed) may legitimately be foregone.

There are two main instruments for advance-care planning: the writing of a set of instructions that record in detail a person's preferences for treatment and care in the future (a 'living will'), and the appointment of a person to whom healthcare professionals can talk when the person is no longer able to talk. It has long been shown that detailed written instructions do not work (Schneider & Fagerlin, 2004). Few people have them; few people can predict their actual preferences accurately; few people can articulate their preferences clearly; and they are often not available when they are needed. In addition, written instructions are not self-explanatory. The course of illness is unpredictable, and a health professional needs to be free to provide good care in the actual circumstances of a patient's illness, as well as when unanticipated circumstances arise: detailed written instructions can privilege past wishes over the provision of reasonable care. In addition, advance-care planning should not focus on an intervention *in and of itself* (antibiotics, say, or the use of a ventilator), but on the use of an intervention *in particular circumstances*. A short course of antibiotics may relieve discomfort in a dying person, and a ventilator may be helpful in an emergency. But each may reasonably be judged to be extraordinary (optional) in the case of a person who is peacefully approaching death. It is better that patients, in advance, identify the person they would trust to do the talking with the health professional when they are not able to do so themselves. And then they should be encouraged to give that person some guidance, for making decisions for someone else at the end of life can be both difficult and distressing.

There are legitimate concerns about advance-care planning. On the one hand, it can reinforce a reductive approach to ethical issues in medical treatment and care at the end of life, reducing an approach that recognises the complexity and sensitivity of a discussion about options for care, that examines the matter from the perspective of the patient, that asks those who know the patient to adopt their viewpoint and to decide what they would have wanted, to an approach that focuses merely on the common law obligation to respect refusals of treatment. No doubt these two ideas – the notion that an intervention can be optional and the common law's notion of the obligation to respect refusals – have developed hand in hand. No doubt they point in the same direction: that the decision is ultimately the patient's and not the health professional's. Nonetheless, today there is a widening gap between them. From the Christian perspective, it still makes sense to talk of treatment that *should be accepted* (for instance, a ventilator in the circumstances of a ruptured appendix). But it would be almost unthinkable for any health department policy to talk of treatment that *should* be accepted: the so-called 'principle' of autonomy tends to dominate everything else that is said.

Nonetheless, advance-care planning can be useful for ensuring both that the proper goals of medical treatment inform the care of people who become unable to make decisions about their own treatment, and that the means used to seek those goals reflect their judgements. Depending on how it is used, advance-care planning can be at worst a stepping stone in policy shifts towards legalising euthanasia and assisted suicide, or at best another way by which to recognise the plurality of values – solidarity, care, compassion, respect for the proper decision-making responsibility of the individual – that ought to inform the care of dying people, particularly those who spend the last part of their lives in hospitals and nursing homes (Dubler, 2008).

Conclusion

Justice in the provision of medical and nursing care to people whose lives are drawing to an end poses both practical and ethical challenges for Australians. This discussion has focused on the ethical challenges, in particular how the requirements of justice in the allocation of healthcare should be understood quite generally and in relation to those at the end of their lives. It has been argued that there are several different ways of understanding what is owed to others, as a matter of justice, in healthcare allocation; that there are several different ways of identifying *who* that other is; and that the idea of 'advance-care planning' provides a useful prism for analysing how best to ensure that, as a matter of justice in the provision of health and aged care, those who are nearing the end of their lives have genuine choices in the treatments and forms of care that we guarantee for them.

Reflective exercises

16.1 This chapter presents four main approaches to justice in the distribution of healthcare resources.

- Summarise each of these approaches, noting the key aspects that distinguish this approach from the others presented.
- Are there any groups within society that may be advantaged or disadvantaged by any of these main approaches? Consider this question across the lifespan of the human person – from the beginning to the end of life.
- For each of the approaches, identify in your current practice examples of such resource allocation, first in general provision of care and then at the end of life.

16.2 With a focus on affirming the dignity of the human person, which approach most successfully achieves this? What is the basis for your answer?

16.3 Essential to the Catholic Health model of care is the Golden Rule of healthcare. What are the key characteristics of this model and the particular applications for end-of-life care? Are there any benefits or limitations to this model of care in palliation of the dying?

16.4 Describe what the chapter presents as the goals and means proper to healthcare. Do you agree with the statement that there is only a *prima facie* duty to preserve life?

16.5 Is it ethical to 'treat' a patient at the end of life? Consider this question in terms of futility, and ordinary versus extraordinary treatment.

16.6 The chapter presents a discussion about advance directives and what justice requires at the end of life.

- What are some of the benefits for the patient and the family in planning care for the end of life?
- What are some of the limitations to advance-care planning instruments?
- In relation to the ethical principle of justice, what are the key elements to ensure that there is 'just care at the end of life' for your patients?

Note

1. These four approaches are distinguished and explained in Fisher (1994). This chapter owes a great deal to Fisher's ground-breaking work. The best published summary of Fisher's work is found in Fisher and Gormally (2001).

References

Aristotle (1976). *Nichomachean ethics*, trans. J. A. K. Thomson, introduction and bibliography Jonathan Barnes (rev. ed. with notes and appendices H. Tredinnick). Harmondsworth: Penguin.

Buckle, S. (1991). *Natural law and the theory of property: Grotius to Hume.* Oxford: Oxford University Press.

Catholic Health Australia (2001). *Code of ethical standards for Catholic health and aged care services in Australia.* Retrieved 20 April 2014 from <http://www.cha.org.au>.

Daniels, N. (2008). *Just health: Meeting health needs fairly.* Cambridge: Cambridge University Press.

Dubler, N. (2008). Tell me about Mama: Facilitating end-of-life decisions. *Bioethics Outlook*, 19(4): 1–8.

Dworkin, R. (1981). What is equality? *Philosophy and Public Affairs*, 10(3): 185–246.

Engelhardt, H. T. (1986). *The foundations of bioethics*. Oxford: Oxford University Press.

Finnis, K. (1980). *Natural law and natural rights*. Oxford: Clarendon Press.

Fisher, A. (1994). The principles of distributive justice considered with reference to the allocation of healthcare. Unpublished PhD thesis, University of Oxford.

Fisher, A. & Gormally, L. (2001) *Healthcare allocation: An ethical framework for public policy*. London: Linacre Centre.

Locke, J. (1975). *An essay concerning human understanding*, ed. P. H. Nidditch. Oxford: Clarendon Press.

Nozick, R. (1968). *Anarchy, state and utopia*. Oxford: Blackwell.

Rawls, J. (1971). *A theory of justice*. Oxford: Oxford University Press.

Schneider, C. & Fagerlin, A. (2004). Enough: The failure of the living will. *Hastings Center Report*, 34(2): 30–42.

Singer, P. (1979) Rich and poor. In P. Singer, *Practical ethics*. Cambridge: Cambridge University Press.

—— (1994). *Rethinking life and death*. Melbourne: Text.

—— (2009). Why we must ration health care. *New York Times Magazine*, 19 July.

Sulmasy, D. (2008). Advance directives as an extension of the tradition of foregoing extraordinary means of care. *Bioethics Outlook*, 19(2): 1–12.

Tobin, B (2002). Editorial. *Contemporary Nurse*, 12(3): 209–12.

—— (2008). More talk, less paper! *Bioethics Outlook*, 19(3): 1–7.

Williams, B. (1985). Which slopes are slippery? In M. Lockwood (ed.), *Moral dilemmas in medicine*. Oxford: Oxford University Press, pp. 126–37.

Index

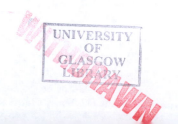